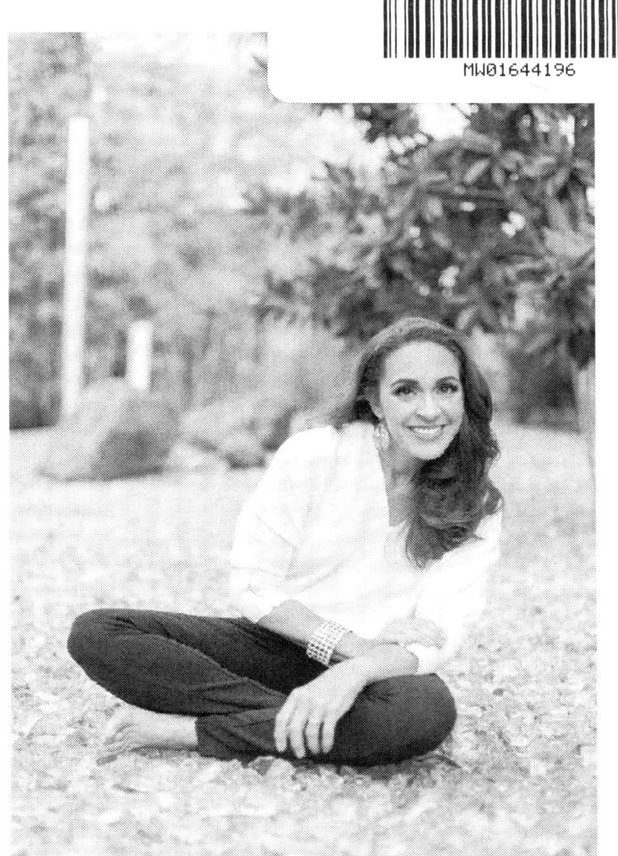

I'm **Dr. Myrelis Aponte Samalot**

I invite you to enter **Homeostasis**

Embrace the change!

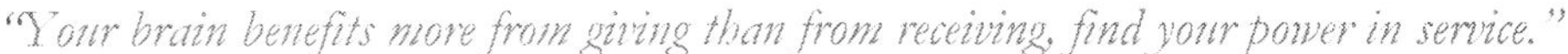

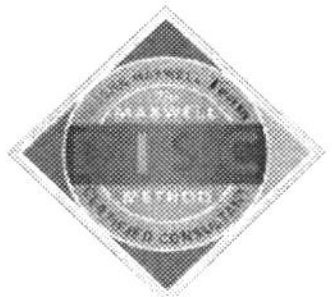

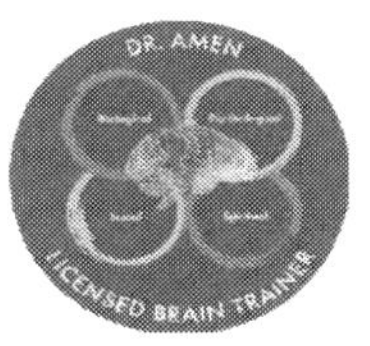

HAPPY BRAIN, HAPPY LIFE

"Your brain holds the 3 keys to a balanced life and homeostasis".

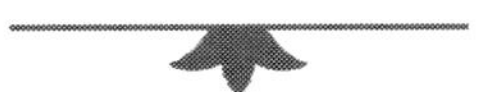

FirstEdition: 2022

ISBN: 9798836599386

Address, editorial design, cover: **Juliana No**
Editing and proofreading: **Juliana No**
Photography: **Juliana Rangel Photography & Denee Hickman**
Translation: **Brayant Manrique & Daviana Alfonzo**

Artwork and vectors:

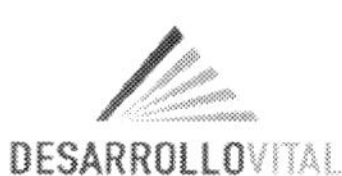

https://www.freepik.es/vectores created by rawpixel.com
https://www.freepik.es/fotos e ilustration created bye freepik
www.freepik.es

Cell phone/ Text 787-529-1584
https://desarrollovital.com/ https://dramyrelis.com

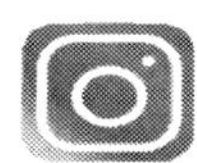

https://www.instagram.com/dra.myrelis/

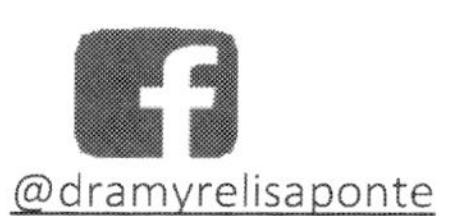

@dramyrelisaponte

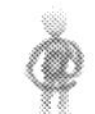

dramyrelis@desarrollovital.com

Content

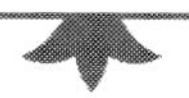

Happy Brain, Happy Life

YOUR BRAIN HOLDS THE 3 KEYS TO ACHIEVE A BALANCED LIFE

"Practical guide for reflection and self-analysis".

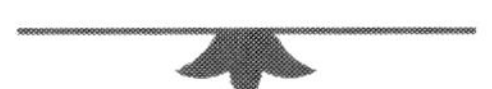

This book and guide is for women to develop a full, balanced and harmonious life. Homeostasis is defined in this text, by Dr. Myrelis Aponte Samalot, as the physical, emotional and social stability and balance that women need to develop their potential in the United States and around the world.

Dra. Myrelis Aponte Samalot

Dedications and Acknowledgments

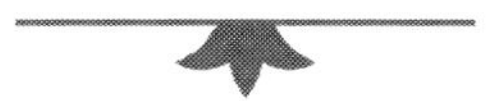

I dedicate this book to my husband Mike Hernandez and my daughters Victoria and Valeria Hernandez. For years, they have watched me dream of writing a book that awakens the potential in other women who, like me, do not give up in the face of challenges and yearn to inspire other women to reach their full potential. Over time, they have seen me support so many people on their path to success and have given so much of themselves to support me in this adventure.

Mike, thank you for your love and unconditional support. You have never let me give up and have always been the one holding my arms up in times of growth.

Victoria and Valeria, thank you for sharing Mom with so many others. Thank you for being my reason for being and for inspiring me to share how much I have learned from you.

Mami and Israel, Papi and Elba, thank you for the blessing of loving me unconditionally. Thank you for modeling moral and ethical values and allowing me to dream and believe that I could achieve great things in life. You taught me from a young age, as I do now with my daughters. Thank you to my extended family and friends for being my most loyal supporters.

Thank you to my mentor, Dr. Lourdes Allen for being a great woman. You inspired me and believed that writing this book and guide was possible and necessary. You didn't let me give up and you shared your beliefs and empowered me along the way. This book is part of your legacy, through me. I infinitely thank the Lord my God for putting you in my path. It is an honor to have the privilege of sharing the stage with you.

Preface

How are you? I'm Dr. Lourdes, mentor of Dr. Myrelis, who is the author of the book, *Homeostasis Your Brain Holds 3 Keys to achieving a balanced life.* "A practical guide for reflection and self-analysis.". I assure you that the contents of this book and guide will positively change the way you view yourself and others, and thus improve your quality of life in the United States and around the world.

I would like you to stop for a minute and ask yourself, what does it mean to be a woman? This question may seem silly, but it really isn't. In the age in which we live, even the most basic conceptions of daily life are being changed or distorted. But, for the purposes of this book and guide, a woman is an individual who not only possesses the anatomy and physiology of the female gender, but also assumes the roles of the society in which she belongs. Pay close attention! The anatomy and physiology of females is extremely wonderful but complicated. Our genital organs, supported by a perfect mix of hormones, give us the capacity and power to create life and form families. In our bodies lies the key to human procreation.

Unfortunately, despite all these achievements, contributions and advances, women throughout history and in all countries and cultures of the world have been and still are considered inferior to men. For example, today women pilot transatlantic flights.

It was not long ago that two women made repairs on the International Space Station, one of the most difficult and dangerous jobs in the world. However, hear me out, it was only a year ago that women in Saudi Arabia were granted permission to transport.

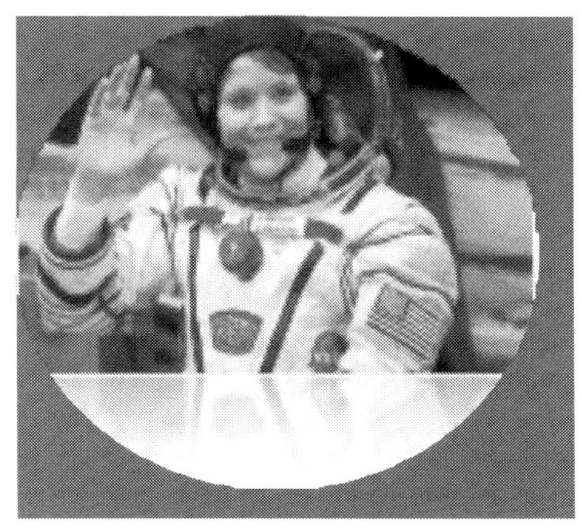

Currently, the government of India is drafting laws that prohibit the annihilation of girls at birth. Newborns of the male gender are welcomed and those born with the female gender are exterminated. In many parts of the world being born female is almost a disgrace!

Women, even in the most developed countries, continue to be victims of mental, verbal or physical abuse in their homes and sexual harassment where they work. Even in the most advanced countries, where women generally enjoy greater freedom and opportunities, there is what is called the "glass ceiling". In a male-dominated world, women may be perceived as too weak or incapable of dealing with the challenges and demands that come with top leadership positions. In other words, despite being procreators and great contributors to the progress of humanity, we continue to face immeasurable challenges around the world, including in the United States of America; especially if in addition to being a woman, you have a profession. Professional woman come to this country determined to reach her full potential and determined to achieve a higher quality of life, not impossible goals, but difficult to achieve when you are a woman.

Did you know that 18% of the population of North America is Hispanic? In other words, approximately 60 million of those residing in the United States emigrated or are descendants of people who immigrated from different countries in Latin America. Of those 60 million, half of them are women. We represent a large population! We are also very unique because we are not only united by language and culture, but we also share the desire and hope to achieve a high-quality life in the United States and in the world. We have also left our countries, cultures, families and all that was familiar to us in search of a better future for ourselves and our loved ones. Therefore, it is my opinion that the challenges women face outside of their country are greater and more complicated than the challenges of others.

And why do I say this? Professional Hispanic women must achieve proficiency in the English language without losing our proficiency in the Spanish language. We have to learn and adapt to the culture without forgetting who we are and our roots. Many of us play multiple roles, including being mothers, wives, and daughters. Most women work outside the home to provide for the needs of the household, as do men. And, to complicate matters further, many of us face racism, discrimination, negative notions and attitudes toward Hispanics, and - most of all - an anti-immigrant spirit that permeates freely in the culture of this country. Pay attention to what I am about to say. If you and I, and all women living abroad, do not take care of ourselves, we can easily fall into depression, suffer from anxiety and see our health deteriorate. Worst of all, these barriers and challenges can prevent us from achieving our dreams and fulfilling the responsibilities that lie on our shoulders. Simply put, depression, anxiety and physical exhaustion, among many other ailments, threaten the health of women today.

It's time to react!

We have to learn and implement strategies that help us or give us the ability to reach our full potential and live high-quality lives. But this, my dear friend, can only be achieved if we learn to live healthy lives. But the health that I am referring to and that we need so much requires, or rather demands, that we live balanced lives. We need to achieve a balance or a state of ***homeostasis*** in all areas of our lives. It is for this, and many other reasons, that my colleague, friend and sister in faith Myrelis, better known as Dr. Myrelis

Aponte Samalot, decided to write the book and guide that you have in your hands today.

A professional in the area of Clinical Neuropsychology with years of experience as a therapist, counselor, public speaker and teacher; above all she is a professional, mother and wife. Dr. Myrelis, through her long career, and from her own experience as a woman, fully understands the challenges we face and how hard it is to live balanced lives. I am confident that this book and guide will give us the knowledge and strategies we need to achieve the balance, or homeostasis, that we urgently need to live healthy lives and achieve the goals we have set for ourselves.

Long live women!

Introduction

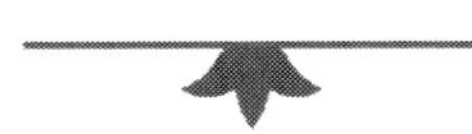

Who could have imagined it! It has been 20 years since I offered my first workshop to a very diverse group of people. How time flies! Over the years I have served employees of public and private corporations, businessmen, entrepreneurs, teachers, fathers, mothers, religious and community leaders. But there is something that has always struck me, how women have stood out for their leadership and commitment to their various roles.

The Latina woman has stood out in her desire to succeed, to work hard for her family's livelihood and for her ability to do diverse tasks to find a balance or equilibrium in her various facets. Over the years, I realized that I could offer virtually the same in all my seminars. Regardless of the topic, I always offered my audience the same three keys, physical, emotional and social health, to live balanced and fulfilling lives. That is why this book and guide is based on years of experience, exploration and discussion with thousands of women on health, wellness and how to achieve a full life in today's world.

You and I know that life is not perfect and no one is perfect. Who we are today is the result of our circumstances, experiences and decisions throughout our lives. It is for that reason that this book and guide is based on the information I have gathered to date. Therefore, it is impossible to pretend that one book and guide has the answers to all your questions, isn't it? My hope is that Happy Brain, Happy Life will be an instrument of change and that it will serve as a guide to provoke new mental paradigms and take steps or actions that will improve your quality of life.

This tool will help you look at the different angles of life and put the weight on the lasting things. I want you to internalize how much your life is worth and how important it is to take care of and develop your physical, emotional, and social health. I will be discussing various exercises and strategies that will allow you to evaluate your experiences and set new goals. As a result of what you will learn in this book and guide, you will be able to establish a plan of action and develop a better lifestyle.

I should add that the value of the teachings and strategies you will find become even more important as it is being published in the midst of the Coronavirus Pandemic (COVID-19). There have been other pandemics in the world throughout history, but never one that has "brought to its knees" the physical, economic, emotional and social health of all humanity. COVID-19 paralyzed the world and took by surprise the big and the small, and the rich as well as the poor. This virus has not respected gender, race, culture, religion or the country we live in.

It has attacked us all equally! However, during and after this worldwide plague, Happy Brain, Happy Life will provide you with the knowledge, tools and skills you need to achieve and maintain a balanced and fulfilling life. The three keys I will present will guide you to physical, emotional and social health, now and for the next 100 years.

The Wonder of Being a Woman

I don't know if you were raised in your home country or if you have been in the U.S. for most of your life, but like me,there are some factors that stand out to us. According to a *Nielsen* article in *Latina 2.0*, published in print in New York in 2017, *"Women have become power brokers in the United States."* In this article they call us the *"catalysts of entrepreneurship and development."* They call us this because of our focus on being fiscally conscious, possessing cultural influence and having a family direction.

I would like to share with you some characteristics that distinguish us as woman. I hope you can see yourself in this mirror so you can begin to see the impact you have on everyone. Did you know:

- There are 165 million in the United States. In other words, we are approximately 50% of the population in the US.
- Women preserve more traditions.
- How wonderful!91% of women who have graduated from high school are enrolled in college, which is not surprising to me.
- Women are very well connected on social media and are more influential.
- Women who own their own businesses, a grew of 87%, double that of men.

I love to see that we are a *catalyst*, since, by definition, a catalyst is an accelerating component of a reaction or result. How awesome! We are agents of change, progress and family togetherness.

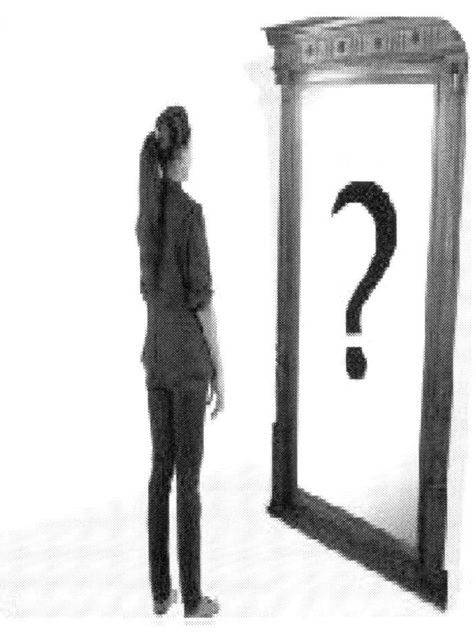

It is with this perspective of today's woman that I long for you to take a good look in the mirror and place yourself in the context of the three keys we will discuss in this book and guide. I want you to join all women who set the example with our leadership and influence. It is my hope that you will also become a role model for other generations of women who come after you.

Homeostasis

If in this book and guide we are going to talk about the 3 keys to living a balanced life, I want to share with you a new term or concept that you can use for this purpose. To achieve balance in any area of your life, it is important to emphasize that you need to develop balance and stability. That is why I use the concept of ***homeostasis*** as the basis of this book and guide.

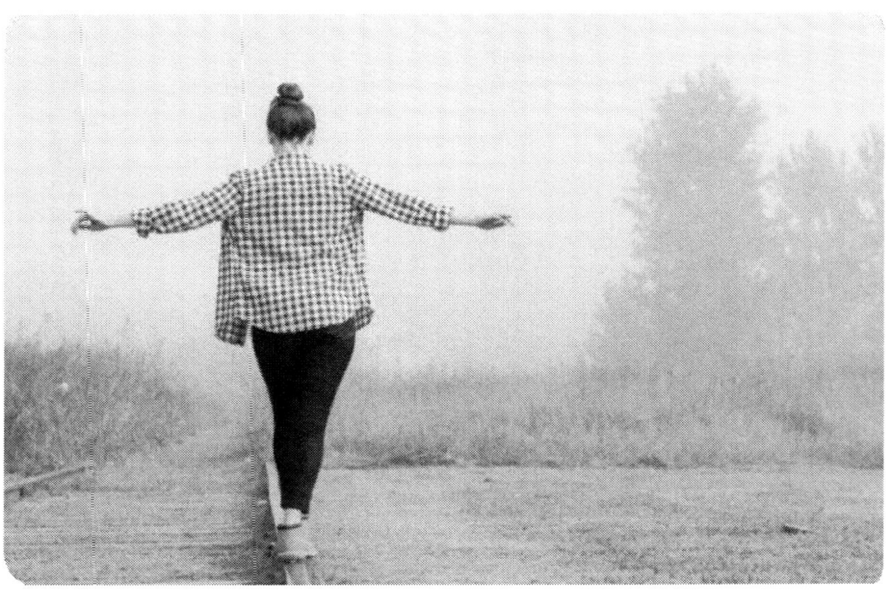

Homeostasis is a scientific term that arises from the Greek words meaning "equally" and "stable". It is defined as the tendency to maintain a state of stability and equilibrium among various elements. I define the term homeostasis in this book and guide as the ability to have stability and balance in and between our physical, emotional and social systems.

We will start with:

HOMEOSTASIS MECHANISM

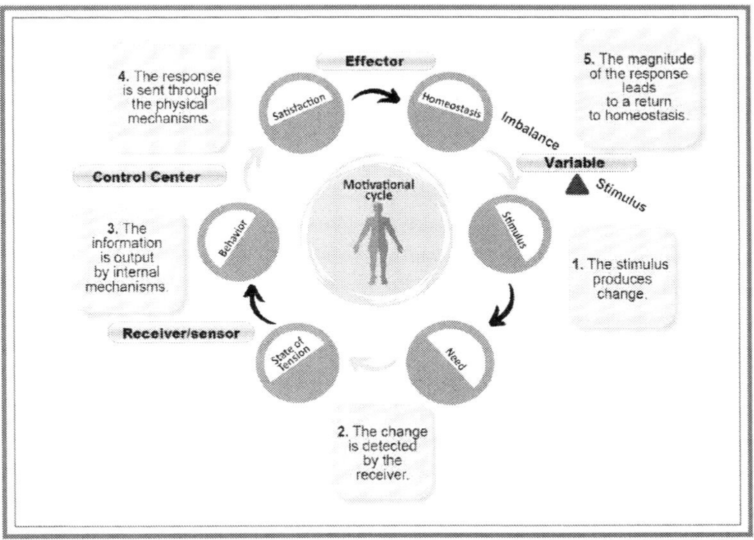

In order for you to understand how human beings, and specifically women, function, I want to pause to talk to you about *Maslow's Pyramid of Needs.* This psychosocial pyramid shows us that human beings are not able to move towards a goal or a high level of fulfillment if they have not been able to meet their basic and physiological needs.

Some of these basic aspects are the needs of our body. These include nourishment, hydration, personal care, sexuality, and rest. These are aspects of being human that we often ignore how important they are. In these chapters, I intend to explain to you three keys that comprise the fulfillment of these needs in a satisfactory manner.

MASLOW'S PYRAMID

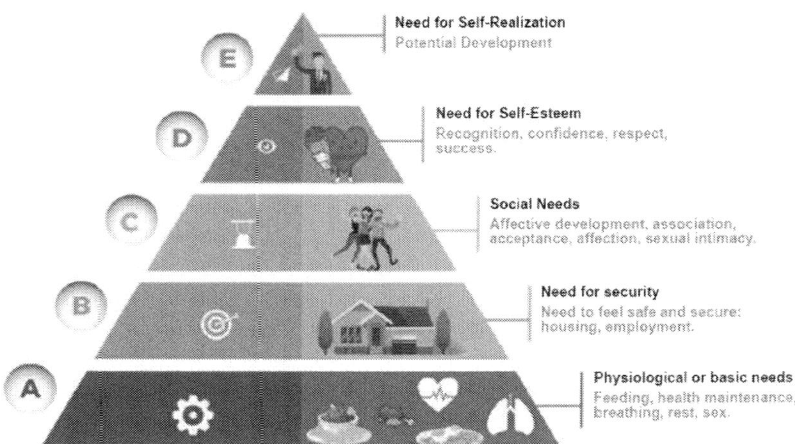

In this pyramid, you will notice that, in order to achieve the need for self-realization or the development of your potential, it is necessary to have addressed four important areas of life. **In the first stage of achievement is the achievement or balanced satisfaction of physiological and bodily needs**. What does this mean? That our body is receiving what it needs to be balanced. Ignoring this stage prevents us from moving or progressing to the next stages. It is for this reason that the base of *Maslow's Pyramid* occupies the most space in the balance of physiological needs.

The second stage of *Maslow's Pyramid* indicates that to achieve self-actualization is related to our need to feel secure. In other words, that our needs for protection and shelter are met. Throughout our lives we have encountered circumstances contrary to our will, which have affected our sense of security. These traumatic experiences have been assimilated and interpreted by our brains, negatively impacting our need to feel safe.

This stage includes the level or quality of affection, love and understanding you received from your parents. It also includes the way in which they provided for you to ensure your survival, such as a place to live, clothes to wear or a school to educate you.

If you somehow lacked one or more of these needs, it is possible that your brain and way of thinking have been affected and, therefore, impaired your development.

I have good news! In this book and guide you will find keys to help you move forward.

The third stage of the pyramid includes more abstract aspects such as life experiences and interactions with people we have lived with over the years. For example, education, socioeconomic environment, values acquired through parents, family and the environment in which we have developed. According to our survival states, it is possible that these stages have defined our path.

When we reach the fourth stage we are considering and understanding psychological factors such as self-esteem, self-image and self-concept. It is here that your personality takes definition and shape. It is at this stage that you can identify whether your experiences have led you to be a leader or follower. Unfortunately, at this level is where many women have stagnated because they have been defined by the negative circumstances of our world or personal lives.

We have finally reached the fifth stage. The most interesting and I want you to pay close attention to it. It is here, where we break the mental paradigms created in the previous stages that prevent you from reaching your self-realization. The following chapters will help you understand where you have come from and how you have been formed; and, above all, will give you the ability to take the necessary steps to rebuild your own pyramid and reach the optimal stage of self-realization. That is where you will enjoy a full and balanced life.

A Practical Model

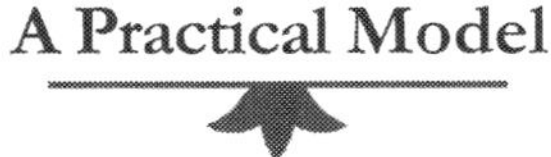

Using this principle as a foundation, I have taken the *Biopsychosocial Model* as the theoretical basis for the three keys we will be studying. There you will realize that, although the name sounds complicated, the concepts are simple and easy to understand.

THE *BIOPSYCHOSOCIAL* MODEL

The *Biopsychosocial Model* presented here considers three important components of our life. First, I will cover the needs of our physical body and discuss some of the basic, but indispensable, elements that promote women's health.

If we go back to *Maslow's Pyramid* that we have just covered, the physiological needs of the human being are the first weapons of defense. When our physical body is not in balance, then we are unable to pay the necessary attention to other areas of our life that require attention and change. That is why, in the first part of this book and guide, I focus on the first key which is your *Body Intelligence*. Both you and I must know our physical bodies and the physiological needs that demand attention to keep them in balance and in optimal functioning. Achieving this body balance will allow us to focus on the next two factors.

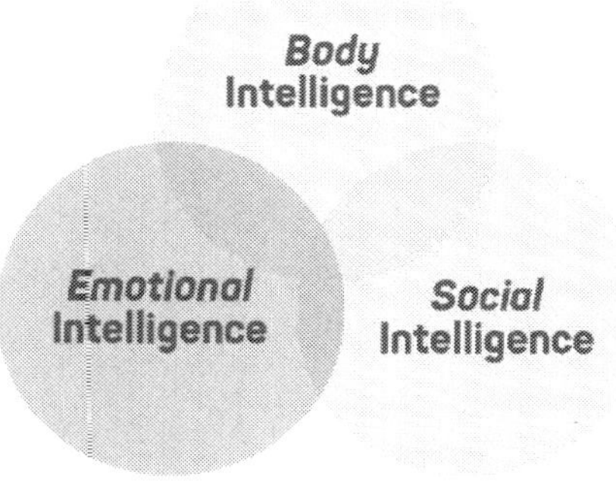

The second key is *Emotional Intelligence* which is the psychological factor. As human beings, we are dominated by what we have learned and our behavior is a reflection of the previous experiences we have undergone since our childhood. In fact, to be specific, since our conception. Therefore, in this second part we will focus on the patterns of learned behaviors and those that we have developed according to our lived experiences. I will also cover aspects of *Emotional Intelligence.* Not only will I define this concept, but I will also share effective strategies to strengthen your ability to overcome adversity and find solutions.

The last part of this book and guide will focus on the third key, *Social Intelligence*, which are the social aspects that make up the third part of the *Biopsychosocial Model.* The fact that we live in a progressive, capitalist economy has diversified our roles in society and in our communities. Our fighting spirit has helped us to take on each role with strength and nobility. In this part of the model, I will talk about our various roles and their importance. I will talk to you about how the experiences we live through allow us to take a leadership role and influence within our family, professional and community circles. And finally, I will discuss the importance of you and me leaving a legacy in life, which is my favorite part. As Dr. Lourdes mentions, "Sooner or later we will leave for the afterlife. But as women, we can contribute with tools to a better world for the next generations."

As you can see, *Body Intelligence*, *Emotional Intelligence* and *Social Intelligence* are the 3 keys to achieve a balanced life or the *homeostasis* that you and I need. May this journey that you started take you through your bodily, emotional and social needs and that it gives you a new perspective or paradigm and the possibility of making changes leading to a higher quality life.

1

PART

TAKE CARE OF YOUR BODY-BRAIN

"A wise man (woman) should realize that health is valuable.".

"If someone desires good health, they must first ask themselves if they are ready to eliminate the reasons for their illness. Only then is it possible to help".

Hippocrates

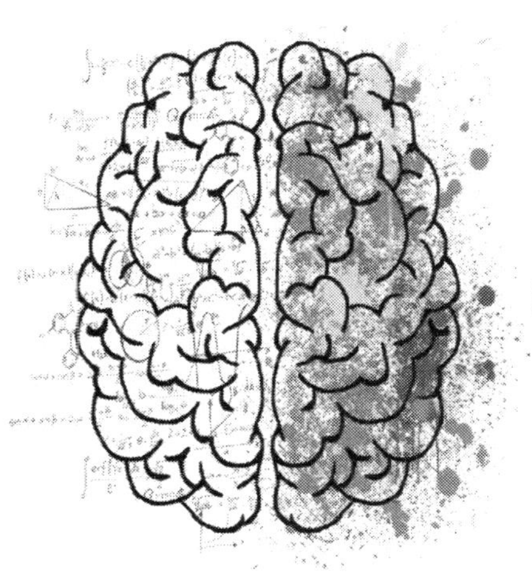

Brain-body = health

CHAPTER 1

Your Body Intelligence

Female Anatomy

I want you to close your eyes for a moment and think about your body. Breathe deeply through your nose and exhale through your
mouth. With your eyes closed, think about the parts of your body that you can notice and which have been the ones that concern you the most. I know you are there, in that moment where we look in the mirror and think of all the physical things we could improve or even change. Or maybe you don't even want to look in the mirror anymore because you think there is nothing you can do.

Typically, you think about the outside first, but stop for a moment and think about your inner self. Feel your body in silence. You may even hear your own heartbeat. I'm sure that, even once, you've felt them in the silence or perhaps in your sleep. It is the best way to know that you still have life and that blood is flowing in your veins.

That is where I want to start. Your body is your most precious instrument and without it you would have no existence. That's why you need to stop at this first key and discover the wonders you can achieve no matter your age.

It is possible that, if you are already in your 30's or older, you have started to feel changes in your body even to stay in shape. What you eat already affects

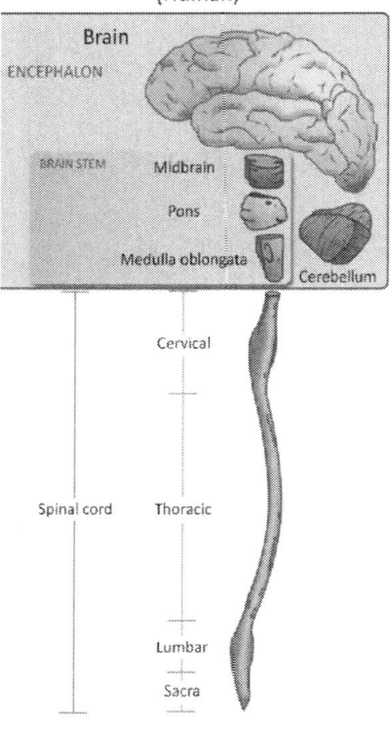

you much more and you spend hours looking for home remedies to have more energy and less fatigue. In this chapter I want to share with you some details of our anatomical and physiological nature that make us unique and that, in turn, play a big role in these changes.

It is important that you spend time getting to know your body, because only in this way will you be able to use strategies that are of greater benefit to you.

As we saw in *Maslow's Pyramid*, the first factor or component is to fulfill or satisfy the needs of our physiological and anatomical nature; in other words to know how the body works. Our body is composed of essential anatomical structures.

Therefore, it is important to evaluate how it works. The first and most important system is our central nervous system, which is composed of the brain and spinal cord. These are the primary anatomical structures, since, without these structures, there would be no presence of life. Therefore, it is important to evaluate their functioning.

¿Are you awake and alert, can you breathe, are you able to ingest food, drink and swallow? Then it means that the basic structures appear to be functioning well. That does not mean that they are in homeostasis - balanced and in *equilibrium* - but I will describe this later.

However, there are anatomical structures that distinguish us as women. First of all, we were genetically determined to be women because our genes are defined or classified as XX. This is something we can in no way change or alter. The genes then give way to a physical anatomy in which we observe that we have internal organs that define us as women. These include: the ovaries, the uterus and the womb.

We are, between male and female, the only ones who can produce and carry a life in the womb, at least up to this point. How wonderful! Likewise, we have an external anatomy that also belongs to our unique anatomy. The breasts and vulva are the external organs that show that we are women.

Each of these anatomical structures requires an internal and external balance for proper functioning. Our nervous system is in charge of ensuring that, as long as we are alive, the parts of our femininity function actively.

It is important to consider some aspects that can affect our body such as genetic predispositions. For example, there are people who have hereditary conditions that physically affect their bodies. On the other hand, accidents or diseases can also affect the anatomical structure of the human body.

The important thing here is to be aware of which systems are in a "normal" state and which, for some reason, are affected. The degree of awareness and acceptance will be important to understand the rest. Therefore, analyze your physical body at this time and become aware of all its parts. Use this guide, for your notes. Think of three areas of your physical body that you wish to improve. Write down some of the symptoms that may be bothering you in your daily life. For example, if as a child you fell off your bicycle and hurt your right knee, it is possible that today, after many years, you have a problem using that knee.

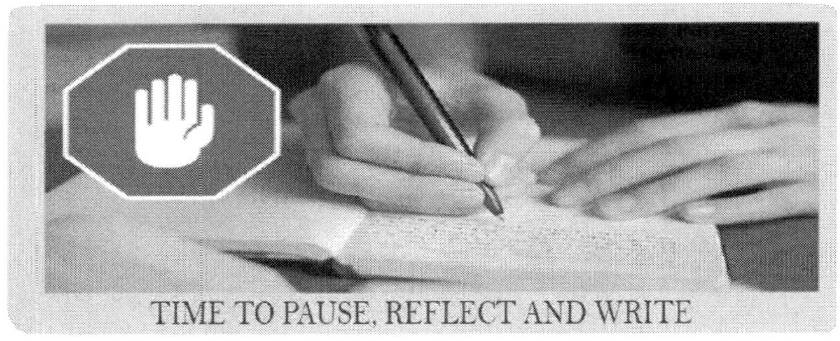

Exercise to Develop *Body Intelligence*

I want you to pause for a moment to think about and write down the answers to the following three questions.

1. What three areas of your body do you want to improve?

____

____

____

____

____

2. What actions will you take to improve them?

____
____
____
____
____
____
____
____
____
____
____
____
____
____

3. When will you take these actions?

____
____
____
____
____
____
____
____
____
____
____
____

Intercellular Communication (Body Chemicals)

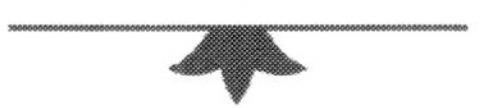

Within the biological component, we need to consider other areas that are not based solely on our physical anatomy. I am referring to the chemistry of our bodies. Yes, those chemicals that we know as our *hormones*.

Likewise, we will consider *neurotransmitters*, or what we call the chemicals that interact at the brain level. These are responsible for our physical, emotional and social responses. How wonderful the human body is! In this section, I will describe some of the most important chemicals that we must maintain to achieve a balanced body.

What do you consider to be chemicals? It is important to remember that the chemicals and *hormones* in our body are directed by our brain. In other words, the **brain** is the first and major precursor to your chemicals and *hormones*. You have various glands around the body that promote the release of chemicals, not only for brain functioning, but for our physical functioning.

We will begin by considering the pituitary gland, as it is the gland that secretes various hormones that allow us to function on a daily basis. The other two extremely important glands are the thyroid and the ovaries. It is these three that work together to produce or facilitate the balance and *equilibrium* that our bodies need to function properly.

What I mean is that chemicals initiate or generate an interaction between the various substances in your body, and through your cells. This interaction of substances enables the ideal functioning of the body. However, when these chemicals are not in balance or *homeostasis*, women can experience somatic reactions, that is, physical or bodily reactions caused by chemical imbalances.

Some examples of these physical reactions can be: exhaustion, fatigue, depressive symptoms, lack of motivation, and many symptoms very similar to the emotional ones. This works this way because the chemicals in your body have an impact at the brain level, even if they are triggered by glands outside of your brain. Therefore, hormones and the organs that produce them coordinate hormonal and many other functions.

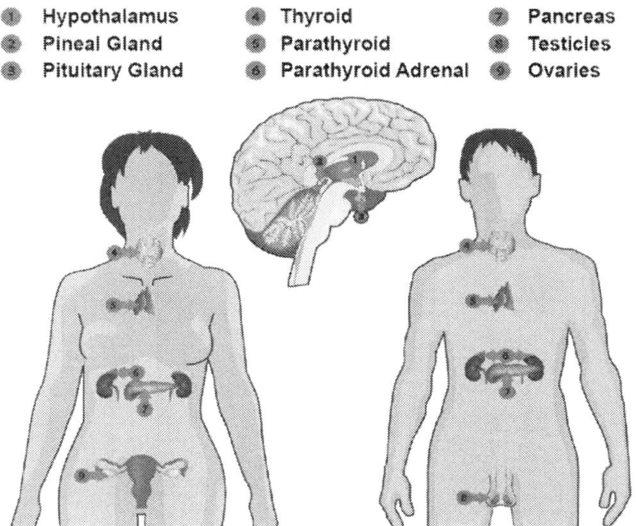

Have you heard of adrenaline? I'm sure you have. When we are stressed or tense, the body produces this substance. Adrenaline:

- travels through the blood,
- produces an increase in the heartbeat,
- dilates the arteries,
- activates pulmonary ventilation.

What it does is to prepare us for a high energy output and that is why we produce it when we are in a tense or dangerous situation. Adrenaline helps us to flee from difficult circumstances or to face sudden and dangerous challenges. Like adrenaline, there are other chemicals in our body that are transported by the blood to all the tissues of our body.

Continuing with the topic of chemicals in a woman's body, I would now like to tell you about the endocrine system and its importance. This system has nine organs that produce hormones. These organs are the endocrine glands. Of these, the pituitary gland (also called the hypophysis) is the most important because it produces hormones that stimulate the other glands.

ENDOCRINE SYSTEM **GLANDS**

In the image you can see which are the glands of the endocrine system. Some disorders and other alterations are produced by the effect of the decrease of a hormone called estrogen.

These alterations or disorders are associated with stages or changes in health such as:

- loss of bone mass (osteoporosis)
- vaginal dryness,
- cardiovascular diseases such as myocardial infarction.

It is of utmost importance, as a woman, that you understand that the balance of your body's chemicals is key or indispensable to daily performance or functioning. Even changes associated with a stage of your life, such as menopause, can be brought into homeostasis. In other words, everyone can live full and balanced lives.

Think about your brain, did you know that it is continually doing work, not only physically, but intellectually, emotionally and spiritually? It is obvious that, from time to time, both you and I feel unbalanced, don't you think? We are going to notice this primarily in the emotional area.

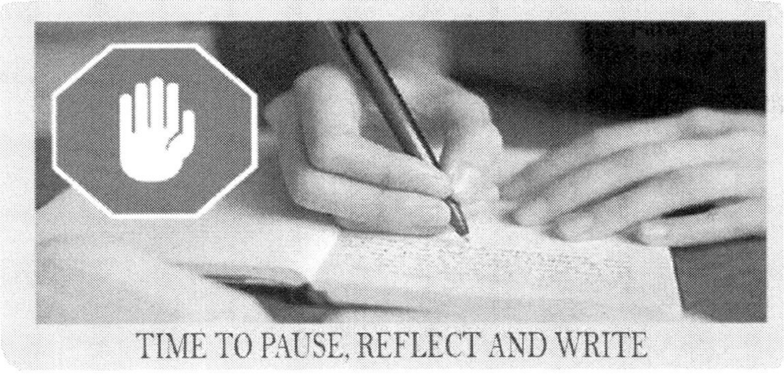
TIME TO PAUSE, REFLECT AND WRITE

Exercise to develop *Body Intelligence*

Pause to ask yourself how you are feeling. Use the following list as an example and check yes to those symptoms that, for the past three to four weeks, you have been feeling frequently. You can also write down.

SYMPTOMS	Yes
Lethargy	
Weakness in the legs	
Tiredness	
Cardiac Agitation	
Fatigue	
Headaches	
Dizziness	
Skin Dryness	
Sweating	
Hair Loss	
Nausea	
Temperature Changes	
Menstrual Cycle Changes	

SYMPTOMS	Yes
Lethargy	
Little or No Sexual Desire	
Other	

I must make it clear that in no way do I intend for you to self-diagnose. Never! That would go against my professional practices. What I want is for you to take responsibility for your body. I want you to learn to listen to it and understand it so that you can more clearly express your needs to your doctor.

For us to truly understand how the chemicals in our body work, we must first understand that every cell in our body seeks to keep itself in balance at all times, even when we sleep. That balance is achieved through the constant exchange of chemicals and energy.

Your cells are like a membrane. What is a membrane? Imagine you have a piece of cloth and you put it in the middle of water, it obviously gets completely wet on both sides. However, every chemical has or does not have the ability to pass through those fabric fibers.

In order for both sides of the cell membrane to have the same concentration of chemicals and for there to be equilibrium, there must be an exchange of chemicals and energy on both sides of the cell membrane. It is our role and responsibility to keep them in balance. Lack of balance at the cellular level manifests itself with unwanted symptoms.

On the other hand, these unwanted symptoms are our first line of defense. Symptoms let us know that our body is not in homeostasis, they are like an alarm that demands immediate correction. It is imperative that you and I get to know our bodies and become aware of its changes.

To provoke *homeostasis* in the cells it is important that you pay attention to the four strategies that I will share with you in the next chapter. These strategies will help you achieve not only chemical balance, but also body balance.

I assure you that these are strategies you can start applying today! But before moving on to the next chapter, I hope you have completed the previous exercises. That way you will know your body better, understand and achieve the balance you need.

Physical Nature
(Intercellular Electricity)

Let me first talk to you about your physical nature. This is where I ask you to please keep an open mind.
I will not talk to you about philosophies that are outside our anatomical and physiological nature. We are beings, not only physical, but intellectual and spiritual. It is for that reason, that as long as we are in this world, we need to understand how the *physics* of our body works.

There are many who want to distort the nature of what our faith is. But science has had the opportunity to discover that our cells are connected through not only chemical interactions, but also electrical interactions. So, when I mention the word *physics*, I am referring to the electrical connections that exist between our cells.

It is possible that when you were little you took a science class where you learned about neurons or brain cells. Our bodies are made up of millions of cells that make up parts of our many systems. For example, we have a digestive system, a cardiac system and an endocrine system, and each system contains cells designed to meet specific requirements in order to function.

As I explained earlier, chemicals are the key to the functioning of cells. However, in order for these chemicals to pass through the valves that exist in the cell membranes and run through our various systems, they need energy. This energy is the *physics* I am referring to.

This energy that exists in the membranes allows the valves in the membranes to open and close. This opening and closing of valves allows desired chemicals to pass through and blocks unwanted chemicals. Some valves need less energy and other valves will need more energy. Without this energy, the valves will neither open nor close. Energy is indispensable for our bodies to work in accordance with chemical balances.

When we understand this connection between the biology, chemistry and physics of our bodies, we can understand the importance of the four strategies I will be sharing with you. Our cells are unable to move chemicals through our bodies without the use of energy. Period!

In fact, the ability to stand, sit and move depends on our energy level. Therefore, I am not talking to you about a mystical energy but the energy that exists in our bodies, at the cellular level, and allows us to live. Without energy we could not even breathe. Now, one of the objectives of this book and guide is that you achieve the ability to increase the energy level of your body.

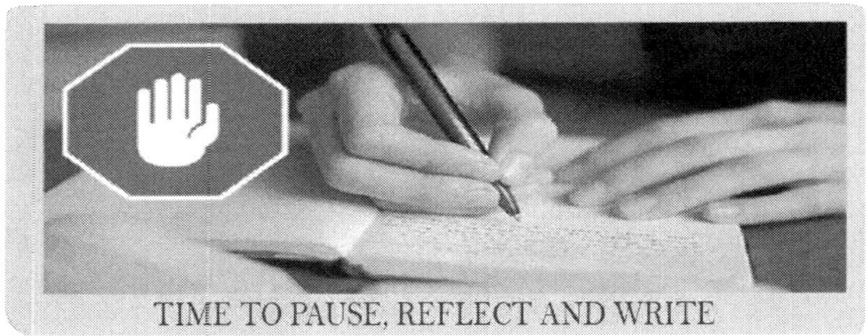

Exercise to develop *Body Intelligence*

Now that you have learned about your biological, chemical and physical needs, it is important to write them down to complete the A-B-C exercise.

A stands for **appreciation.**

So, I want you to look at yourself and appreciate how you see yourself. Now I want you to express yourself honestly - fearlessly, this book and guide are yours!

____

____

____

____

____

____

____

____

____

____

The **B** stands for **blessing**.

Notice that blessing is nothing else than "to bring bliss" or "to fill something with bliss". Therefore, write something that fills you with bliss about your physical body and your health.

____

____

____

____

____

____

____

____

____

C stands for commit.

What will you commit to in order to improve your overall physical health? Make a list of the steps you will take to improve the integrity of your physiology or chemistry.

____

____

____

____

____

____

Always remember...

To Appreciate

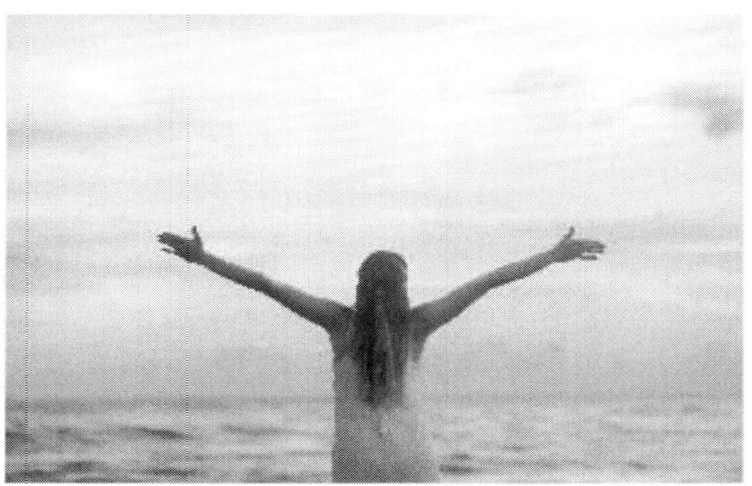

To bless

To commit yourself

CHAPTER 2

Strategies for Body Homeostasis

When our lives are balanced, the body's energy levels should be functioning properly, in order to accomplish everything we desire. That is why each of the following strategies is key, no matter how simple they may seem. For me it is important that you can see their value, because they will help you live a balanced life.

1. Hydration (H2O)

Let's start with the first strategy, hydration. Our cells are made up of approximately 70% water. Most people don't know that most of their bodies are made up of water, yes pure water. Humans can sustain themselves without food for several days. However, without water we can die quickly. This is one of the requirements for keeping our cells in homeostasis. Water is key to that balance.

I imagine you have heard many theories about how much water we should drink. Although every culture has a different belief regarding the amount of water we should consume, science has taught us that in order to maintain the proper level of water in our bodies, we should ingest certain amounts.

PERCENTAGE OF WATER IN THE *HUMAN BODY*

There is a practical formula for how much water would be ideal. However, this formula is not the only thing that determines how much water our bodies should consume. I will talk about this later.

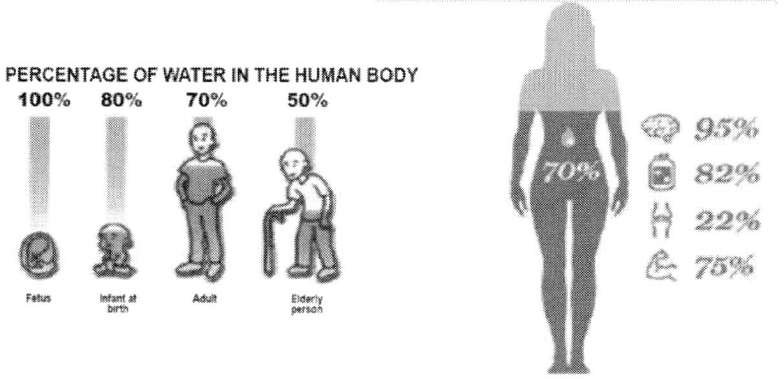

For example, when our bodies retain water, we might think that we should limit our water intake. However, our body has the ability to "flush". A toilet, for example, is not the most beautiful image I can present to you.

Of course, it contains dirty water! What do you do to make the toilet flush the dirty water and fill up with clean water? In Puerto Rico, my country, we say, "Baja la cadena" (Flush it down). We lift a chain that allows more clean water to go down and, therefore, that momentary drop of water allows all the water that was dirty to go down and disappear from the toilet. So do our bodies. One of the most effective ways to achieve homeostasis is by ingesting water on a regular basis, especially when we are stressed.

When you are stressed or have worries, the water you drink has the same effect of flushing. Stress causes hormones and neurochemicals to build up in your body that overload your frontal lobe. This is the part of the brain you use to think and coordinate your actions.

In times of stress, our frontal lobe has a very difficult time paying attention, focusing or making decisions. When we drink water, these neurochemicals are balanced and suddenly, you feel refreshed, liberated, and with a greater ability to think and make decisions. See? Water has the same effect as a "flushing".

In fact, the European Hydration Institute teaches us that water:

1. It is important for proper brain function. When you are hydrated your brain receives more oxygenated blood and you are able to stay alert.
2. Adequately consumed, it is essential for the kidneys to function well, helping them to eliminate waste and unnecessary nutrients through urine.
3. It improves the digestive tract, since water is necessary in the dissolution of nutrients so that they can be absorbed by the blood and transported to the cells.
4. It is a great ally of the skin, helping it to maintain its elasticity and tone.
5. It acts as a lubricant for muscles and joints to function properly

The question we should ask ourselves now is: how much water should I drink? According to the *National Academy of Sciences, Engineering and Medicine*, adult women's water intake should average 2.7 liters (11.5 8-ounce glasses) of water. Now, 20% of this water is already consumed through meals.

It would be logical to understand that a person who weighs 150 pounds should drink less water than one who weighs 257 pounds. To get a more accurate number, we must first calculate our weight in pounds and divide that weight by sixteen (16). The result of that division is the number of glasses of water you should drink per day. Let's not forget that each glass is 8 ounces. For example, a woman who weighs 158 pounds should consume approximately 10 glasses of water per day.

Be very careful, in the United States they use 16, 18 and even 20-ounce glasses, especially when we ingest sugary drinks with no nutritional value. That is one of the main reasons for the exaggerated level of obesity. Don't worry, all the water I suggest, you should not consume at the same time.

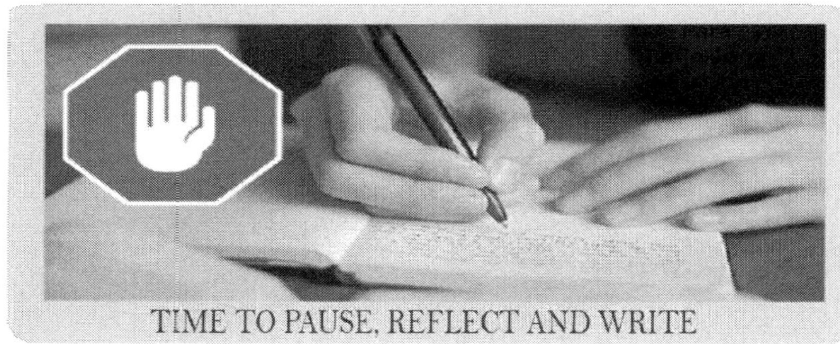

Exercise to develop *Body Intelligence*

Now I want you to calculate the amount of water that, according to this formula **(Weight ÷ 2 = Volume in ounces of water)** you should drink. Then compare that amount with the amount you are currently drinking. What can you conclude?

____

____

____

____

That amount of water you calculated is what you should increase, little by little, until you achieve it. Increase 1 glass every couple of days and you will see how, in a short time, you will have trained your brain to do it automatically.

Drinking water when you feel thirsty is good, but it is a sign that you have gone past the right time. When the body feels thirsty it is because it has a great need for water; it is already out of balance.

Where I currently live, in Florida, the weather is extremely hot and humid. Horseback riding is a sport that requires a lot of stamina and oxygenation. When I started training, I felt that I was not able to perform the full time of the lesson, I ended up reddened and sometimes even almost dizzy.

Until one day the trainer told me, have a glass of water before you start.

I said to myself: that's right! I don't know how I didn't think of it before. When I started drinking water before I started everything changed, no more dizziness! Therefore, to feel balanced, it is important that you drink water constantly and, above all, before exercise.

In your critical or stressful moments, it is important that you consume the full eight ounces, not just a sip. It is at that precise moment, those eight ounces of water will help you reach the balance or *homeostasis* that your body needs to think well, focus, and make the right decisions.

2. Nutrition

The second strategy for developing *body intelligence* that promotes balance involves nutrition. Nutrition is not just about eating well. Good nutrition must include a number of key nutrients so that the chemicals in our bodies are balanced.

Now, there is a very important aspect to this line. Nutrition is not only about what you eat, but, depending on your lifestyle, may require supplementation. Today we have access to numerous food alternatives that do not provide nutrition. For that reason, creating awareness of how to eat right will help us develop our *body intelligence.*

I want to share with you some changes that, although small, have improved my health and, therefore, my quality of life. These changes are my favorites, I practice them every day and they have not altered my eating style too much. As small as they may seem to you, I assure you that if you put them into practice, it will improve your eating habits.

Let's start with the type or kind of plate you use to serve yourself. Have you ever thought about it? You must change the way you eat. No matter how nice a plate looks to you, if it is big, you will put more food on it than your body needs. I always use a smaller container or plate to avoid serving myself exaggerated portions.

In many occasions our depending on the generation and culture we may have been told us: "the fatter you are, the healthier you look and too thin must mean you are sick". However, those extra pounds or being overweight, over the years, negatively affects our health. I will never forget when my grandmother Carmen would see a grandchild or relative, she hadn't seen for a long time, and she would say, "How cute you look with those extra pounds!" In those days, being chubby or plump was fashionable and was a reflection of being healthy, but what did Grandma Carmen know about cardiovascular conditions, arterial problems, cerebrovascular disease, among others? Today, people have the possibility of having a long life because of the knowledge that exists about how to take care of the body and this includes how you eat.

I want you to consider how much of what you eat provides benefits to your body. Today, there are so many types of diets that I don't want to convince you of one or the other. Whether you eat meat or are a vegetarian, the important thing is that you eat a balanced diet so that on a cellular level you are balanced.

You must also pay close attention to the amount of carbohydrates and sugars you consume. Coming from a Hispanic background foods, although delicious, are high in carbohydrates and, consequently, high in calories. It is for that reason that women, more than men, suffer from cardiovascular conditions such as high blood pressure, high cholesterol levels and diabetes. Our problem is not that we eat poorly. Our problem is that we don't eat right. Please serve yourself smaller portions and decrease the amount of carbohydrates and sugars you consume; your brain will be happier.

The Decade of Changes

Now, I want to share with you some tips for those like me who are past 30. If you are in your 30's or earlier,

I just ask you to read carefully and prepare yourself. Most women think it's too late to change their bodies or improve their health. Although prevention will always be the best remedy, preparing your body for changes is even more important. This is how I teach young girls and women of reproductive ages. It's not taking prenatal vitamins when you know you are pregnant, it's taking them to prepare your body, your cells and your genetics for a healthy chromosome crossover. So, this is your time if you are in those stages.

Maybe you are in those years where perimenopause is looming, the period before menopause, which can last from 5 to 10 years. Or maybe you have already entered menopause, the period where you have already gone six months or more without a menstrual cycle. But what should women do to live healthy lives during these stages? Nothing! There is no need to do anything special.

Perimenopause and menopause are important stages in women's lives because they comprise one-third of their lives.

If you find yourself in one of these stages, full of physical and physiological changes, and you want to live in health and balance I advise you to:

- you should eat a diet rich in calcium to prevent osteoporosis. Milk and its derivatives are good sources of this mineral.
- control the use of fats to avoid high cholesterol levels. Use olive oil and exclude lard and butter.
- lower your salt intake to avoid high blood pressure.
- increase the consumption of legumes, vegetables, fruits and cereals. These are rich in vitamins and minerals.
- drink 1.5 to 2 liters of water a day. Dehydration is dangerous and deprives you of energy.
- drink orange, lemon and other citrus juices. These are rich in vitamin C.
- do not smoke or drink stimulating beverages such as coffee and tea. These increase hot flashes characteristic of these stages of a woman's life.
- exercise daily to strengthen your heart and delay osteoporosis.

Let me share with you a reality regarding weight. Although exercise helps us burn calories and therefore lose weight, 70% of the weight we could lose depends on what we eat and how much we eat. This means that, although physical activity or exercise is important, what you eat will determine not only your weight, but also the proper transfer of chemicals and intracellular energy.

Eating the right foods allows us to generate the right chemical exchanges to be able to execute an effective physical activity. What does all this mean that I have just explained? In "rice and beans" (simply put), as they say in my country, what you eat is essential to generate the balance, equilibrium and energy that your body needs.

As for supplementation, there are also several sides. There are clinicians who believe and say that we do not need supplements if we eat well. On the other hand, there are those who say that food supplements are essential, because cooking food damages the nutritional content. Other clinicians warn us of the harm of preservatives in canned or packaged foods. If I go on, I won't stop. There you can see that we are being bombarded by a thousand recommendations.

My dear friend, at the end of the day, it's all about balance. Just as my husband, our daughters and I have learned to supplement our diet daily in a balanced way, without exaggeration. The important thing is that we eat well so that our bodies and our brains function at their maximum capacity.

Happy Brain, Happy Life: Your brain holds the 3 keys to achieving a balanced life and homeostasis. "A Practical Guide to Reflection and Self-Analysis," is being published in 2022, in an era that demands continuous, perhaps excessive, activity. Do you have enough time in the day to do everything you have or want to do? Of course not! To live balanced lives, we need dietary supplementation. I recommend that you use high quality, organic-based supplements.

NUTRITIONAL PYRAMID

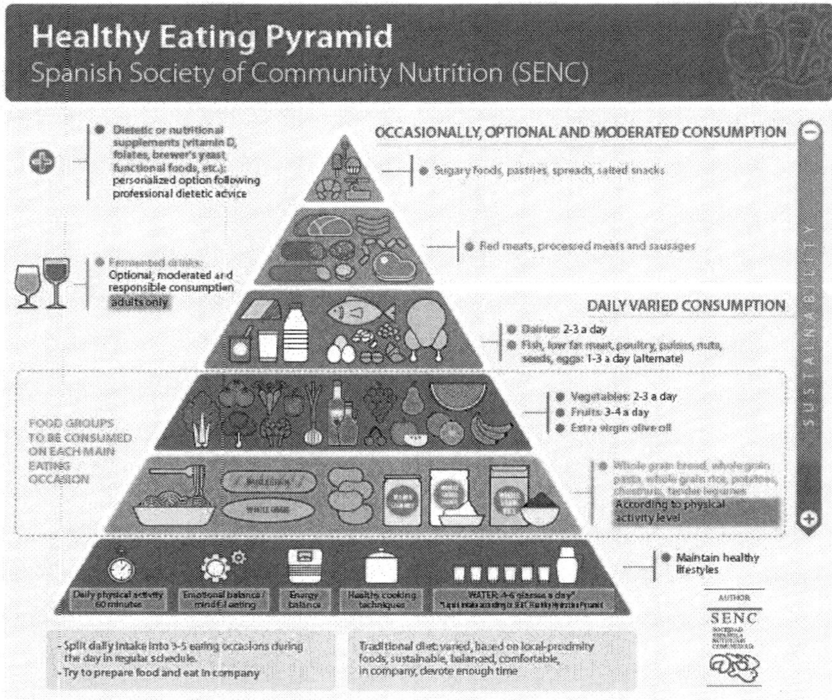

According to the Office of Women's Health (OWH), all vitamins and minerals are important for good health. Vitamins and minerals often work together in your body. Ideally, you should get your vitamins and minerals from different types of foods you eat. Therefore, fill your plate with fruits, vegetables, dairy products, grains and a variety of protein foods to create a healthy plate.

We can also supplement the diet with high quality supplements. In the following table I include the list of supplements that we should consume on a daily basis. However, this should be modified according to your specific needs. It is important that you consult with your doctor at least every six months.

ESSENTIAL SUPPLEMENTS FOR WOMEN

Supplement	Benefit
Folic Acid (Vitamin B9)	• It helps in the formation of blood cells and DNA (genetics) for new cells. • It also helps prevent certain birth defects that occur in the first three months of pregnancy.
Vitamin B-12	• It helps the body produce red blood cells. It also helps your neurons (cells in your brain and nervous system) function properly.
Vitamin D	• Along with calcium, it helps strengthen your bones and prevent osteoporosis. • It also helps reduce inflammation in cells and helps fight disease-causing germs.
Calcium	**Calcium** helps protect and strengthen bones and reduces the risk of osteoporosis. It also helps transmit messages between your brain and muscles.
Iron	**Iron,** forms healthy blood clots that carry oxygen to your body. It also helps form certain hormones and connective tissues in your body.

For more information on dietary supplements, please visit http://www.desarrollovital.com

Finally, exercise caution with recommendations in the various media, including social networks. These are full of alternatives and options, making promises that lead to great frustrations. By making small changes, as I have suggested from the beginning of this book and guide, you will see consistent and permanent results.

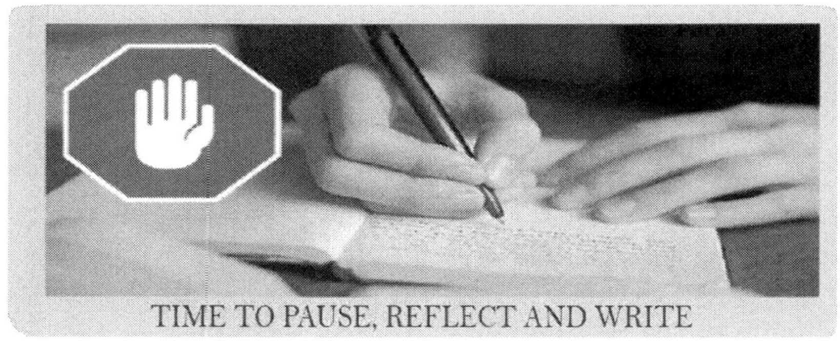

Exercise for developing *Body Intelligence*

It is time to pause and reflect on what we have learned. You are going to write down the small changes you will incorporate into your nutrition and supplementation to improve your physical health and achieve a state of homeostasis.

Now, these last two strategies are mastered by your brain. Don't forget that small, daily, and above all consistent actions will be your route to success.

____

____

____

____

____

____

____

3. Physical Activity

My friend, how much have you heard about the importance of physical activity? I don't know if you remember your adolescence or your childhood. You may have been extremely active or, on the contrary, you were taught that being too active was not appropriate. What does this have to do with anything? When we are children, our bodies create a pattern of activity in the brain that when not exercised does not learn and shuts down.

I remember my mom saying to me, "That girl is white rice," an idiomatic phrase meaning that she was always into everything, I mean, every activity she could find. Not only was I social, but I loved movement. So, I was always into dancing, gymnastics, swimming, horseback riding, acting, among others. Of course, I had those opportunities which I consider a privilege. My body and my brain were always in activity. I need you to see physical activity as a need of your body. And that activity, as I explained earlier, needs a lot of energy. Without energy it is impossible for you to exercise.

Today science teaches us that we must produce or we are the producers of the energy we need. Yes, it is possible to create the right levels of energy for our bodies to function at their peak no matter what your physical capacity. Many women have told me that they can't exercise because they have a bad knee, herniated disc or arthritis. It saddens me to see that they have already given up. If they understood that small changes in their daily activity can have tremendous results, they could improve their health.

I'm not recommending that you go to the gym three times a week for an hour. If you haven't done it so far, you won't do it tomorrow either. What I want you to do is to train your brain to do what you do want, which is to improve your health, right? Your mental paradigm shifts will allow positive changes in your lifestyle. In other words, if you change your thinking, you will change your life as well.

According to the *Colombian Journal of Cardiology*, physical activityprovides multifactorial benefits with effects on the immune, hemostatic, autonomic, metabolic and hormonal systems. These effects, and others, can be applicable at different stages of a woman's physiological history. Let's pause to retrain or reprogram your brain to include or assimilate physical activity as part of your own lifestyle. Physical activity is important for the homeostasis of your cells because:

1. Increases oxygenation of the cells and, therefore, keeps the cells in balance.
2. Stimulates the production of neurotransmitters that provide an experience of pleasure and satisfaction.
3. Strengthens the heart rhythm improving its performance and preventing its dysfunction.
4. Causes energy consumption that allows us to use calories, burn fat and, as a result, lose weight.
5. Decreases the possibility of diabetes or keeps it away for a while.
6. Improves the lipid profile by decreasing cholesterol and triglycerides and increasing good cholesterol.
7. Improves bone quality and muscle strength decreasing the possibility of falls and fractures.

Today, health experts recommend that we exercise 30 minutes or more per day, preferably every day of the week. Physical activity should be of moderate intensity and long enough to expend 200 calories a day. This can be achieved by walking a brisk 2 miles or 3.2 km. With all the technology we enjoy today, this should be easy to achieve.

But the reality is that when we go out to do some kind of exercise, we get fatigued and tired. The next day your brain says, "Girl no, what are you putting yourself through that torture for?" In that instant, your brain won the battle!

Period and it's over!

What I propose to you is very simple and -perhaps- different. I want you to, little by little, get your brain used to it until you reach those 30 minutes. So, start with just 10 minutes. Yes, just 10 minutes! It takes the brain 21 to 30 days to create a new habit. I'm not looking for you to lose 20 pounds in one month - no way! What I am looking for is for you to have lasting results and, for this, physical activity must be part of your daily life. That's why you should start with just 10 minutes a day.

If you are already used to exercising, congratulations. You meet one of the requirements for a long life. If water and nutrition are essential for survival, physical activity is essential to achieve it. This is the plan I recommend.

1. Choose 5 exercises that you know how to execute well. They should be varied, for example:

   a. Jogging in place

   b. Squats

   c. Jumping jacks/jumping jacks

   d. Knee raises

   e. Push-ups (On the floor or to the wall)

2. Use your digital watch or cell phone to set the timer for 10 minutes and do not rest during these 10 minutes.

3. Start with the first exercise for 1 minute and at the end of that minute, move on to the next one.

4. Once you finish all five, you repeat them and that's it, you've finished a 10-minute circuit.

   This table will help you to start the exercises. But remember to always check with your doctor if you can do them.

Mark with an **X** the ones you have been able to complete.

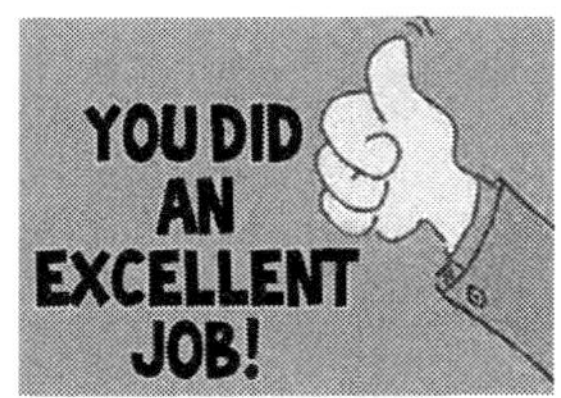

Exercis es	Time 1 minute	Time 5 minutes	Time 10 minutes

The secret is to change exercises just when your brain and body start to get tired. This is how you distract it with the next exercise. What will happen when you try this technique? Many incredible things happen in your brain.

First, because your body is not used to exercise, all your brain and physical systems will trigger cardiac activity and, as a result, you will expend energy and burn calories.

Second, the time you spend exercising is not long enough for your brain to rebel and start complaining. That way, you can easily do it again the next day, until you complete your first month.

Third, you will find that, in just two to three days, you will want to do one more minute and one more minute, because your brain is already adjusting. You will start to feel better because you are seeing the accomplishment and you are producing pleasure neurotransmitters among many other benefits.

10-MINUTE CIRCUIT EXERCISES

FAT BURNING
EXERCISES
Jumping jacks
50 jumps
Jumps Squats
15 reps
Knee raises
15 reps each sidereps
Push-ups
15 reps each side
Lunges
20 reps
Static squat
1 minute

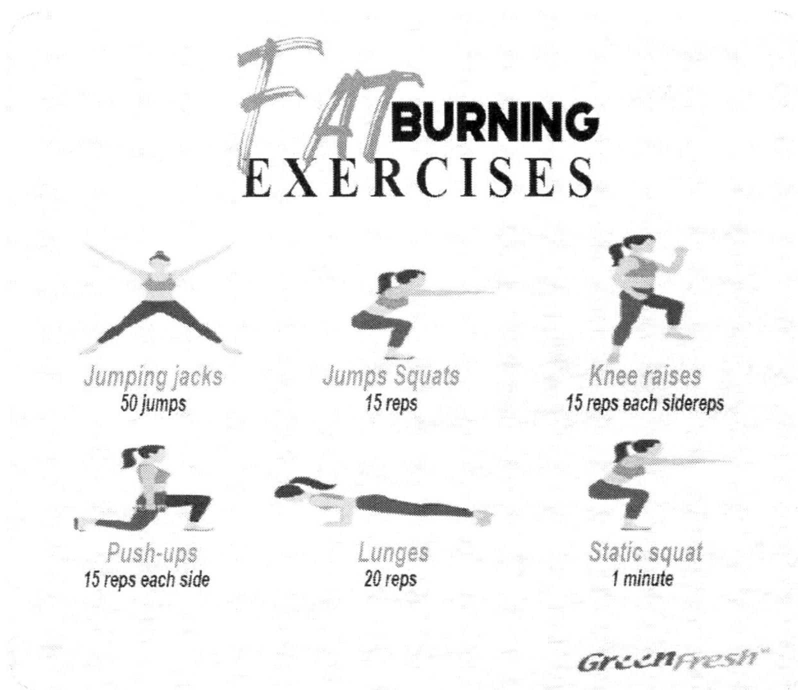

I assure you that after the first week you will feel more confident. I only make a few recommendations so that this method does not fail.

Increase by one (1) minute when your body asks you to, not before. If you get ahead of yourself, your brain will play a dirty trick on you and you will not continue.

Do not go over ten minutes, even if it seems too short, especially during the first week. Later, little by little, you can keep adding minutes so that by the third or fourth week you will have reached 30 minutes. That's when your brain has already created a pattern of daily physical activity.

Don't take rest days during those first three or four weeks. You need your brain to learn this new pattern in your life. If you give up a rest day, the next day you will feel like it was the first day.

Alternate the exercises, to create a little confusion or change in the pattern. This way the brain stays interested and does not get bored with the process or routine.

Exercise according to your body's capacity. There is no need to overdo it. Exercise in moderation. The important thing is that you put in the effort and focus to make it work.

I would also like to add that when you have achieved the pattern and habit of exercising every day for 30 minutes, include other physical activities that you enjoy. Make sure the activities you choose are consistent, close to home or work so you don't give them up. Also incorporate physical activities that may include your partner or children. That way, you get exercise and enjoy the company of your family. For example, you can walk, run, swim, dance or practice any type of sport.

I recommend that, before starting any exercise program, you consult with your doctor to evaluate your health and physical condition. Your doctor will tell you what type and how much physical activity you can do. Nowadays the diversity of exercises or physical activities is immense. Therefore, I am sure that no matter what your physical condition is, you will be able to find a program that is right for you.

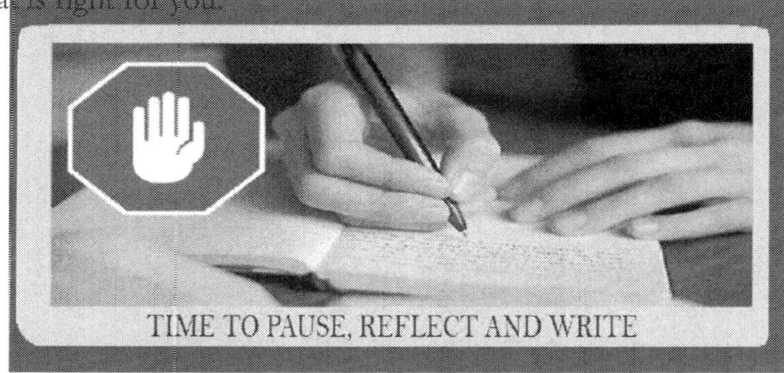

Exercise to develop *Body Intelligence*

It's time to pause and reflect on what you've read. Over the next three weeks I want you to document the number of 10-minute circuits you have accomplished.

Write down how many minutes you have accomplished. Also document how you felt during and after each week.

____

____

____

____

____

____

____

____

____

____

____

____

____

4. The Rest

Rest is a topic we can talk about and share incredible stories about. Especially if you are a mother, wife and professional, your life is surrounded by countless early mornings followed by sleepless nights. Personally, as I write these lines it is 12:00 in the morning. It is at this hour that both my husband and my two daughters are asleep.

I remember when I was a teenager; I slept a lot. I also used to get up late. Our bodies have stages and each one has its own characteristics and needs. I love to seize the day. When I was a military school student, I remember that I would gladly get up at 5:00 a.m. to be ready early. But in the afternoon, when I came home from school, I would take a nap for an hour before I started studying. I no longer enjoy such privileges, but I do understand the reason for that stage and the important role that sleep or rest plays.

My greatest experiences regarding rest did not occur during my university studies. During those years I was still in complete control. The most significant adjustments were when my first daughter Victoria was born. I decided to become a nursing mother and this meant being available to my baby as needed. That is when my long journey of sleepless nights began.

The more days went by, the more my brain was loaded with fatigue. I was looking for every little bit of space and time to rest and recuperate. You can imagine!

During that growing stage Victoria was waking up every 30 minutes. It was not easy. Thank God that my husband, even though he worked, was understanding and supported me as much as he could. But my friend, the reality is that the responsibility we carry on our shoulders is gigantic. I experienced drastic mood swings, anxiety and depressive days. These were times when we didn't know how to overcome them, despite the information and knowledge we both had. What did we do?

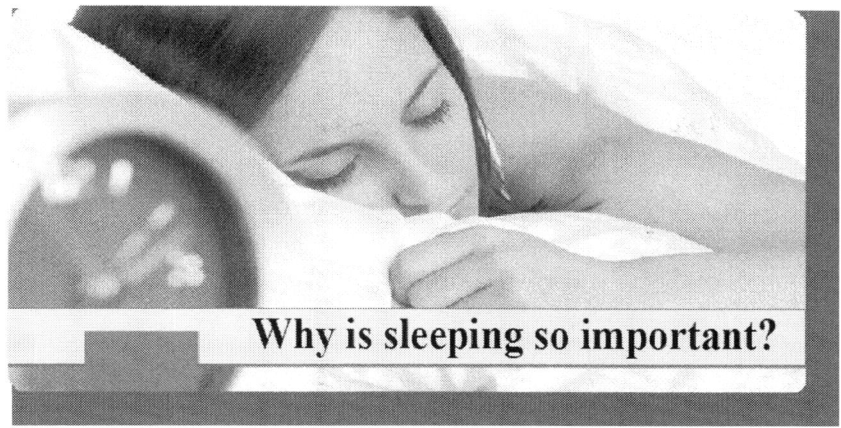

We made the decision to work as a team to achieve positive results. It's experiences like these that make me think about how many women go through similar stages and experience similar circumstances, but are alone or don't know how to share what they are feeling with their partners or family members. It's as if expressing how exhausted they feel is shameful or a sign that they are ineffective mothers.

The recommendations I make in this section are for you to take positive action. There is always a way to improve the quality of our sleep/rest. Don't forget that it's the small adjustments that achieve big results.

I want you to think about all the factors that can interfere or prevent a good night's sleep. Work stress and family responsibilities, even unexpected challenges, such as illness, are factors that can disrupt your rest. At times like these it is very difficult to get a quality night's sleep. Although it is not possible to control all the factors that may prevent you from resting, you can adopt habits that promote better quality sleep. At the National Institute of Health (nih.gov) you can find useful guides and resources to improve this area of your life.

Let me explain some general aspects or characteristics of sleep. When you sleep, even though you are unconscious, your brain and body functions are still active. Sleep is a complex biological process. It helps you process new information, stay healthy and feel rested.

During sleep, your brain goes through five different phases. Different things happen in each phase, such as specific brain wave patterns or patterns of electrical activity in the brain. In certain phases of sleep, your breathing, heart rate and temperature may be faster or slower. It is in stage 5 that rapid eye movements (REM) occur. It is important to know that some of these stages will help you feel more rested and energetic the next day. The different stages of sleep help you to:

- feel rested and energized the next day.
- learn information, make reflections and form memories.
- rest your heart and vascular system.
- release more growth hormones, essential for children to grow.
- increase muscle mass and cell and tissue repair in both children and adults.

- release sex hormones, which contribute to puberty and fertility.
- prevent illness or make you better when you are sick by creating more cytokines (hormones that help the immune system fight various infections).

How much sleep do you need? The amount of sleep you need depends on several factors, including your age, lifestyle, state of health and whether you've been getting enough sleep. If you're an adult like me, you'll need 7 to 8 hours a day.

Some people think that adults need less sleep as they age. However, there is no scientific evidence to prove this. It is true that as people age, they tend to sleep less or spend less time in deep, restful sleep. Older people also wake up more easily. The amount of sleep you get is important, but the quality of sleep is critical.

For example, there are people whose sleep is often interrupted. Some have difficulty going to bed or may not spend enough time in the different stages of sleep. If you have doubts about the quantity and quality of your sleep.

I ask you these three questions and mark with an **X** yes or no.

1. Do you have trouble getting up in the morning?

_______________ **Yes** or ____ **no**

2. Do you have trouble concentrating during the day?

_______________ **Yes** or ____ **no**

3. Do you feel sleepy during the day?

_______________ **Yes** or ____ **no**

If you answered yes to these three questions, you should start sleeping better. If you have doubts about the quantity and quality of your sleep, consult a specialist so that you have the tools to help you improve it.

I want to talk to you more about the negative impact of not sleeping well. Did you know that when you don't get enough sleep you can feel tired? Lack of sleep affects your performance, including your ability to think clearly, react quickly and form memories. This can lead you to make poor decisions and put you in risky situations. People who don't sleep well are more prone to accidents.

Sleep deprivation can also affect your mood. Lack of sleep or rest causes irritability (especially in children and adolescents), depression and anxiety.

Tiredness or lack of sleep also affects or harms your health. Scientific studies tell us that not enough sleep or poor sleep increases your risk of obesity, high blood pressure, heart disease, Type 2 diabetes and kidney disease.

Not getting enough sleep can affect the release of hormones that help you build muscle mass, fight infection and repair cells. In addition, in children it can cause them to not release enough of the hormones that make them grow.

Sleep deprivation increases the effect of alcohol. A sleepy person who drinks too much alcohol will be more affected than a well-rested person. Here are some tools I use that are also recommended by the *Mayo Clinic Sleep Institute.* They are simple tips. Just choose to change one or two of these recommendations at a time and try them for at least seven days. Be patient! Don't forget that your brain has a hard time creating new patterns or routines.

1. Pay attention to what you eat and drink before bedtime. Don't go to bed hungry or feeling too full.
2. Create a relaxing environment or space. Create an ideal room for sleeping. Often, this means a cool, dark, quiet room.
3. Limit naps during the day. Long naps during the day can interfere with nighttime sleep.
4. Incorporate physical activity into your daily routine. Regular physical activity helps you sleep better as long as you don't overdo it.
5. Manage worries. Try to resolve your worries or concerns before you go to sleep.
6. If you work at night, you may need to take naps, keep the lights on in your workplace and limit shift changes to allow your body to adjust.
7. If you often have trouble sleeping, contact your doctor as soon as possible. Although almost everyone, especially women, can have a sleepless night from time to time, it is dangerous not to get a good night's sleep every night.

Remember that the purpose of this book and guide is for you to find that physical, emotional and social balance. Therefore, there are no diets, exercise programs, or magic pillows that can produce long-term results. Temporary results will only bring frustration and listlessness. What is important is that you make decisions that can change your mindset or mental paradigm and empower you to take positive action.

It doesn't matter if you are still in your thirties or if you are past forty. If you are young and healthy, be prepared. If you are no longer young, take immediate action. Start living the best time of your life. What is the best time of your life? Your best time of your life is the time you are in today! You can develop your body intelligence and today is your first day.

Exercise to develop *Body Intelligence*

At this time, I would love for you to pause and reflect on what you have read and write down your answers to the following questions.

1. How many hours of sleep do you currently get per day (on average)

____

____

____

2. What positive sleep habits can you incorporate into your daily routine to improve the quality of your daily rest?

____

____

____

2

PART

GROW WITH PURPOSE

"Elegance is, when the inside is just as beautiful as the outside."

Coco Chanel

"The greatest evil that can befall man is that he should come to think I'll of himself."

Goethe

C HAPTER
3

Your *Emotional Intelligence*

How I think and feel

I wonder where you were when you learned from the media that the COVID-19 virus (Coronavirus) appeared to be a severe version of influenza. Suddenly, we were faced with an invisible enemy. A virus that could be transmitted even by the people you love the most. Everyone is in danger of losing their lives. What a terrifying moment!

We now find ourselves practically locked in our homes. Schools were closed, flights cancelled, and restaurants could only provide services from a distance. Fear and desperation gripped the masses. The last straw came when we could not even buy toilet paper, among many other basic provisions of daily life.

Who would have thought that, in free countries like the United States, we would live through times when our freedom would be impeded by an invisible but lethal enemy? I believe that, in the last 100 years of human history, mankind has never experienced so much uncertainty. It seems unreal, doesn't it? That's why Happy Brain, Happy Life, "A Practical Guide to Reflection and Self-Analysis" will help you achieve a balanced life even in the most difficult circumstances you encounter.

I had to alter my work schedule and adapt to the new reality of remote and digital work. Now, my two daughters were at home all day, and my husband was working from home. In the midst of this crisis, I decided to continue writing this book and guide. Being able to connect with you through these lines was something I couldn't let go.

What did I do? I was able to reflect on the stages of grief which include denial, courage, acceptance, forgiveness and thus restoration. I was able to experience each of these and process them by bringing them to my level of awareness, to acknowledge them and work through each of the emotions and feelings I was experiencing. One of the reasons I was able to process these stages is the time I dedicated to the development of the second key to achieve *homeostasis* or personal balance. I am referring to the key to emotional intelligence or psychological perspective.

You may have heard on many occasions what emotional intelligence is. This concept is defined as the capacity we have to face challenges and be able to overcome them. Daniel Goleman developed this term in the 90's, during the decade called, "the decade of the brain". This type of intelligence is highlighted by a term *resilience*. It is nothing more than **our ability to face and overcome adversity.**

We are all going to go through various difficult moments, traumatic experiences, but it is in you the ability to overcome them. So, let me explain a little bit how this process works in your command center, yes, in your brain. All your experiences have an important place where everything you think and everything you feel comes from.

First of all, both life experiences and genetics are important. Although genetics are relevant, they do not necessarily define you and are the least important. It is the various experiences that make our neurons or brain cells connect. This is how the information from each experience is transmitted and our memories are generated. And, according to the level of relevance or importance of each experience, the information is recorded in short- or long-term memory.

Did you know that experiences are accumulated and generated from conception? Therefore, those experiences your parents lived or those you lived while in your mother's womb may have definitely impacted your way of thinking and expressing yourself.

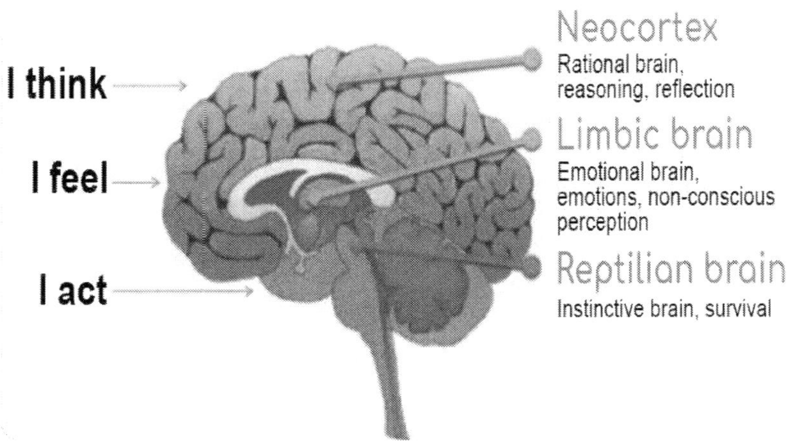

At conception our brain begins to form. The innermost part is formed first, that is the reptilian brain, and then the outer part, which we call the neocortex. If you look at the picture you will see the architecture of the human brain. As you can see, our brain is an extremely large and complex structure. For example, in your brain there are specific areas responsible for the way you think and react to the experiences around you. However, each experience is determined by the level of importance and influence in your life.

As I mentioned earlier, physical and biological needs are primary and basic in the life of human beings. Many times, we do not take care of them well or in the right way and, as a result, we experience negative emotions. Why? Because our brain responds in a defensive way to make sure that our basic needs are met to protect life.

Look for a moment at the next image I am going to show you. Next to the hippocampus is the amygdala.

This small area is responsible for our fear response.

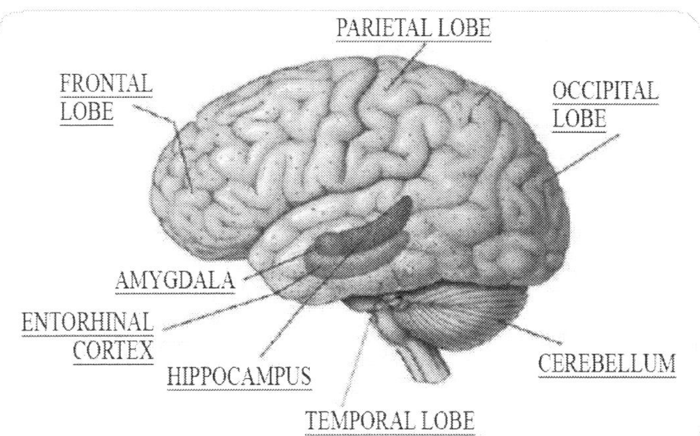

You may have heard that in the face of fear we fight or flight. It is an instinctive response called "fight or flight". This is the mechanism that allows us to protect ourselves from a predator. Not only is it an innate response, but it makes us react according to the experiences we have lived before.

What fears have you developed? What fears have you learned from other influential people in your life? What are you afraid of? I remember when my girls were one and two years old. Their curiosity was greater than their fears; and, although it still is, I can already see the influence of others in their lives. I remember how as toddlers they loved to chase the lizards and find a way to touch or catch them. It was an adventure! They wanted to satisfy their curiosity. But, as soon as they observed other adults reacting with fear, their brains interpreted or assimilated that lizards are to be feared. Now correcting that memory or attitude of fear is more laborious, although not impossible.

Another very important area in our brain is the hippocampus. It is there where experiences are stored in the form of memories.

In the previous pictures you can see that the hippocampus is below the cerebral cortex in order to be protected. It is there that your long-term memories remain and endure. That's why my daughters are still a little afraid of lizards.

All our daily experiences are recorded in the cerebral cortex, the outermost part of the brain. However, those that were extremely important - be they pleasurable or traumatic - will be recorded in the long-term memory, in the hippocampus. We all have difficulty forgetting traumatic events. Similarly, it is very easy to remember events of great joy and pleasure. For example, it is difficult to forget the process of childbirth, since it involves a lot of effort and strong emotions.

You may have difficult memories in your life, such as abuse, rape, or physical or emotional mistreatment. Perhaps you have had painful experiences such as divorce, abandonment or betrayal. All of these experiences, while extremely painful, should not be what marks your long-term memory. As long as you decide to create new memories, you will have the ability to override whatever has been recorded from your previous experiences. But I'll talk about that in a moment.

You should know that our intellectual or thinking capacity is generally shaped by **genetic factors, stimulation, education, practice and life experiences.** I imagine you've already realized that four of the five factors that make up thinking are created by external experiences and information.
Your genetics don't define you, my friend! Our genetic factors, no matter how much "negative" history they have, do not override our life circumstances.

According to the *Theory of Multiple Intelligences*, taught by Dr. Howard Gardner, intelligence is not unitary, it is not one. Intellectual or cognitive intelligence is defined as a group of patterns that measure thinking ability. Gardner explains that there are other strengths, brain skills or aspects of our brain capacity, and among them is *emotional intelligence*. This is the ability to recognize and manage one's own and others' feelings.

Emotional intelligence allows us to respond to personal, family and social demands. It also allows us to adjust emotionally to each situation and gives us the ability to achieve our full potential. That is why the second key to this book and guide is *emotional intelligence.*

I remember when I was 21 and completed my college degree with an incredible energy, capable of succeeding and doing great things. Falling in love started a struggle against my culture, my religious beliefs and who I really was. Although I had not yet found my purpose in life, I knew I was created for great things. What did I do? I chose marriage over a career. By then I thought I had the ability to live a balanced life and the power to maneuver whatever came my way.

I was very brave and self-confident.

I will never forget my father's gesture when I told him I was getting married. He let out a laugh that I still remember. However, I thank him and my mother for allowing me to learn from life. They did not spare me pain. They, within the circumstances, believed in me and let me mature on my own.

To make a long story short, I got divorced 3 years into my marriage. I wanted a career and my husband at the time, although a good person, had different life expectations. I simply knew in my heart that I had been created and destined to serve outside of the family setting to fulfill other purposes.

One of the reasons I had to go through those experiences was not understanding my purpose in life. If you don't find who you are, you can't find ***happiness***. So, my journey of discovery began after a divorce, feelings of rejection, loss, failing, disillusionment. I don't know if you have gone through such experiences, but rest assured I have good news for you, the best is yet to come.

The first concept I wish to introduce to you is your **self-concept**. **Self-concept** is nothing more than what you think of yourself. How do you define yourself? How do you treat yourself? What do you say to yourself? Notice that I use four important verbs to consider, and these are: think, define, treat and say.

How do you think you are? You are pleasant, friendly, generous, nice, loyal, faithful, hard-working, hard-working, enterprising.

How do you define yourself? How do you think of yourself? Are you smart? Do you have abilities? Do you have talent? Friend, the reality is that in many occasions we answer these questions in a negative way, which is unacceptable. This, among others, are behaviors that do not allow us to reach our potential and prevent us from achieving balance or emotional homeostasis.

Loving yourself is one of the most important aspects of a woman's life. Without love for yourself and who you are, you will lack one of the main elements to achieve a good psychological development. However, loving ourselves is something that many of us did not learn as children. At least, we were not explicitly taught it from the time we were little. As children we repeatedly heard expressions such as, "you must be good," "you must brush your teeth," "you must go to school," but not so often were we told, "you must love yourself," "you must pamper yourself," or "you must like yourself." Perhaps, belatedly, we were told, "love yourself, for no one else will do it for you." I know that often confuses you. On occasion women have asked me, "What's that about loving yourself?" Doesn't that sound selfish?

In this section I will also talk about *self-esteem*, and how this concept differs from *self-concept* and *self-image*.

Do all these concepts have the same meaning?

Loving one another is a behavior worthy of praise. However, over the centuries it has also been criticized by society. Some think that those who love themselves are selfish. The image of selfishness has underestimated the real value of *self-esteem* and this has created confusion and misunderstanding. Let us see how our *self-esteem* is formed and what factors sustain it.

First of all, *self-concept, self-image* and *self-esteem* are not the same thing. Although they are closely related, because from my theoretical framework, *self-esteem* is composed or formed with *self-concept* and *self-image*. However, these three are different. In a general way we can say that *self-concept* answers the question, what do you think of yourself? *Self-image* answers the question, what is your opinion of your appearance? Together and well-structured, they shape *self-esteem*. Let's take a closer look.

Self-concept is a term used to designate what you think of yourself. As the name implies, it is the concept you have of yourself. Consequently, this will determine how you treat yourself. In other words, *self-concept* determines what you say to yourself, how you say it, how you demand it of yourself and how you do it. In the face of life's events, you can

mistreat yourself or pamper yourself. If the event is negative, depending on how you conceive yourself, you will give yourself constructive or destructive criticism. For example, if you fail a test you can say to yourself: "I studied and did not pass, therefore, I will have to study more"; or you can say to yourself: "I am a loser". The second is a destructive criticism. In the same way, if the event is positive you can say to yourself, "I passed because I tried hard and I deserve it" or you can say to yourself, "It was pure luck". The second expression is a destructive criticism. The conception you have of yourself, that is, your *self-concept*, will lead you to define yourself in one way or another.

Self-concept is the image we have created of ourselves. It is not only a visual image, since it is rather the set of ideas that we believe define us, at a conscious and unconscious level. This set of ideas includes a virtually infinite number of concepts that could be contained in the image we have of ourselves. In short, each idea can hold within it many other ideas, creating systems of categories.

For example, one component of our self-concept could be the idea we have about our sociability or intelligence.

Do you consider yourself shy or sociable? Do you consider yourself intelligent or incapable of learning? There are a multitude of elements or ideas that are part of our self-image and self-concept and we group them under the same label. In short, self-concept is the set of characteristics that serve to define the image of the "self".

Self-concept is a dynamic process, caused by a mixture of interactions between genes and environment. Therefore, it is not isolated within us, but evolves as a result of our experiences and habits. It is for this reason that the self-concept is closely linked to our social life, which I will discuss in the last two chapters of this book and guide.

I now tie self-concept to **self-image**. **Self-image** is the perception of your physical aspects. How do you see yourself? When you look in the mirror, what do you see?

I should clarify that *self-image* is influenced by a number of factors.

For example, the media, family, friends, culture and society greatly influence the image we have of ourselves. These influences can define how I should be, what I should look like and what I should do.

Self-image is extremely important for a balanced life. If you do not achieve a balanced *self-concept* and *self-image*, you will not achieve a balanced *self-esteem* or a state of emotional homeostasis. Therefore, you must make every effort to achieve emotional balance. Only then will you be able to find satisfaction and pleasure in life.

We recognize ourselves. We look at ourselves and say, "I am beautiful" or "I am pretty". Both you and I have a unique image of ourselves, of how we perceive ourselves physically, regardless of the term beauty. Although social canons and the weight of social comparison influence you, you are responsible for considering yourself more or less pretty or beautiful from a totally subjective point of view. This is your *self-image,* refers to the opinion you have of your image.

The *self-concept* and *self-image*, mentioned above, will largely determine your self-esteem, which will ultimately judge you positively or negatively. Let's not forget that our *self-esteem* also depends on our immediate world, which includes your parents, teachers, friends, family, etc. Our immediate environment, as well as the relationship we establish with the things we experience, develops an idea of how we see ourselves or believe we are.

So, what do I mean by *self-esteem*? We've heard this term a lot. However, you and I understand what triggers healthy *self-esteem*. *Self-esteem* **is the value we place on ourselves based on the perceptions we have of ourselves and the result of our own evaluations**. It is a developmental process. *Self-esteem* is not inherited; it is learned and internalized.

Self-concept + Self-image= Self-esteem

Self-esteem is also directly impacted by our spiritual growth or development. Remember I told you that
we are physical, intellectual and spiritual beings. This is where the spiritual component comes in, essential for balance or *equilibrium* in our daily lives. What I believe about myself is demonstrated in the way I present myself to others. If I do not understand the spiritual value I have in life, much less will those around me understand me.

As I said before, the value we give to who we are is not inherited, it is learned and internalized. This learning is our letter of introduction to each of the things we do and the circumstances we face. It determines our actions, our feelings, our way of relating and our way of doing and undoing.

Success, failure, fear, strength, confidence, insecurity and what we do in all areas of our existence says a lot about our self-esteem. It will be with us all our lives. More than working on it and not letting it play tricks on us, we must take care of it, pamper it and review it.

Self-concept and *self-image* strengthen your own identity. It is a starting point; but *self-esteem* encompasses the totality of your *self-worth*. Your *self-esteem* is as relevant as your own life.
Is it modifiable? Yes, it can be worked on and improved. As your self-esteem improves, your perception of self will improve and you will live your life with more peace of mind, positivity and emotional health.

In short, what I think of myself and the vision I have of myself are the pillars of *self-esteem*. Having a good *self-esteem* brings advantages for our health and psychophysical balance. It is essential for every action, for every feeling and for every step we take.

The frequently mentioned phrase "love yourself, for no one else will do it for you" means that:

1. You accept your mistakes so that you analyze and criticize yourself in a constructive way.
2. You congratulate yourself when you have done something good or of good quality.
3. Modify what needs to be improved in your life without mistreating yourself.
4. Love, cherish and care for your thoughts.

Only you are responsible for doing it. I assure you that when you do, you will achieve greater emotional health.

In the hierarchy of human needs that we saw in the introduction of the book and guide, *self-esteem* is described as the need for appreciation. Appreciation is divided into two parts. The first part is self-esteem, which includes: self-esteem, self-confidence, and self-reliance. The second part is appreciation of others, which includes: the recognition, acceptance, and respect we receive from others. According to Maslow, appreciation is the respect we owe to others, regardless of their notoriety. Appreciation of oneself and others leads to self-actualization.

Carl Rogers, exponent of humanistic psychology, proposed that the root of many people's problems is that they despise themselves and consider themselves to be worthless and unworthy of being loved. In fact, the concept of self-esteem has been approached since then in the humanist school as an inalienable right of every person, synthesized in the following sentence – "Every human being, without exception, by the mere fact of being human, is worthy of the unconditional respect of others and of himself; he deserves to be esteemed and to be esteemed. You are worthy of esteem and to be estimated".

We all have a mental image of who we are, what we look like, what we are good at and what our weaknesses are. We form that image over time, starting in our childhood. You have already generated your own mental image.

Much of your self-image is based on your interactions with other people and your life experiences. This mental image has contributed to your current self-esteem.

Now, remember the story I told you. Those experiences were the result of what I learned from a very young age, as I grew up in awe and respect of our Creator. I sought that spiritual guidance by being part of a religion. However, I was not cautious as I believed everything I was told. I passed up opportunities to grow intellectually because I was taught that I was created to be a missionary and get married. However, this was not in line with my dreams, nor with my expectations. There came a time when the influence of others was so strong that I agreed to those beliefs. That was the moment when I got married. You saw how that part of my story culminated. Up to that point, I was unaware of how much my, "me," who I really was, had been shaped by social, cultural and religious influences.

No one was responsible for me putting my dreams aside. I was responsible. As the years went by, I realized how I had allowed others to define or influence the development of my self-concept and self-image, and thus my self-esteem. The beauty of it all is that I learned that emotional intelligence is learned and developed. So that is what I did in the years that followed. I dedicated time to learn and develop my emotional intelligence.

I managed to have the ability to break with the religious paradigms I had in my mind. Thus, I opened my thinking to true spiritual opportunity, which is born out of a relationship between the Spirit of God and myself. It is a relationship that goes beyond following a spiritual leader or belonging to a religious organization. It is the relationship that exists, or should exist, between the Spirit of God and your spirit, intellect and body. That relationship empowered me to understand the image I was created in and the capabilities I was given. I was created in the image and likeness of God and empowered to fulfill my purpose in life. I was created for great things!

My dreams should not have stopped at that stage of my life. It was then that I decided to take up my dreams and my goals, recreating my life and starting over.

As you can see, my life story includes a divorce at age 23. Yes, divorce is painful. Getting divorced is a loss steeped in self-doubt, guilt and rejection. I married young believing it was the right thing to do. Despite the pain, it was at that moment that I gave myself the opportunity to create a new life of new horizons and full of opportunities. In addition to accepting great losses, I had to experience pain, abandonment and rejection. By accepting my situation, I began to find myself. I was stronger than I thought I was. It was then that I decided to throw myself into the adventure of a new life. I began to learn that life is full of opportunities, and that all the tears shed before would pay off in the future.

After several years I achieved a professionally very fruitful life. Still, there were some personal goals missing in my life. At that time, I thought that, if I were to marry again, I would probably not have children; but my spiritual being knew that there was much more ahead of me.

It was almost 13 years of searching and waiting. Only when I was mature enough to have a new opportunity did it appear. During all those years I was growing in many other areas of my life. I grew as a leader, as a businesswoman, as a professional and as a person. In those years I also learned to value having a family. And that is when God rewarded me with two new opportunities, a great partner and husband and being the mother of two beautiful girls, Victoria and Valeria to love and take care of for the rest of my life.

I don't know what your story is. I only know that whatever your *self-esteem* is at this moment, it is only the fruit of your past, and that today you can learn and develop a healthy *self-esteem* that generates new options in your life.

As women living around the world, I can see how racism, language, cultural change, economic limitations and economic limitations can all take a toll on your self-esteem. Maybe you feel that you had a career in your country and now you can't pursue it. You feel that, because you don't speak English or another language, you can't progress. You feel alienated from your children because now they only want to speak English. It could be that "machismo" reigns in your home. Friend, I assure you that everything you have experienced and continue to experience has negatively impacted your self-esteem. Let me tell you that to achieve the balance or *homeostasis* you deserve and need to make the decision today to learn, grow and develop a self-esteem that will lead to a ***happier*** and higher quality life for you and those you love.

Explore your talents, study the language, develop a business, strengthen your image, strengthen your spiritual life and, above all, connect with other women like you. All of this can and will transform your life.

So now get ready, as I will share with you some of the strategies that helped me during all these years of personal growth and transformation. I know that some of these tools will help you achieve the emotional homeostasis you so desperately need.

These strategies that you will learn have been very effective for many of my clients. Which ones you choose or use will pretty much be part of your style and what goes with your beliefs. I also want you to take the challenge to be an emotionally strong person, because you can. This is your time to develop a balanced emotional intelligence.

You can do it!

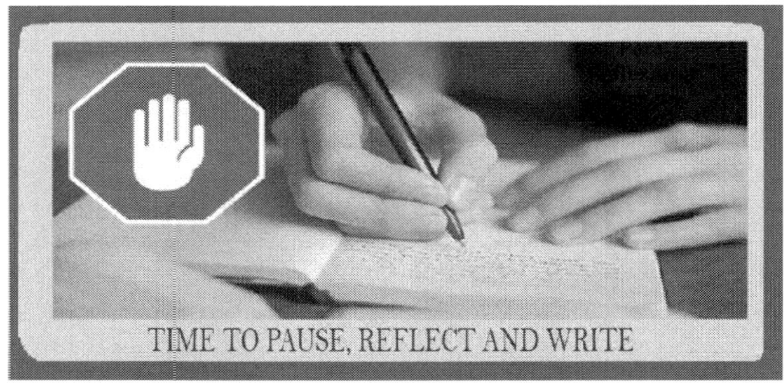

Exercise to develop *Emotional Intelligence*

Since we have seen the differences between self-concept, self-image and self-esteem, and how these three are related, it is important that we do the A-B-C exercise. Express yourself sincerely, but with love for yourself.

No fear, this book and guide are yours!

Since the letter **A** is the first letter of the word appreciate, write something for which you are appreciative to be.

____

____

____

____

____

____

B is the first letter of the word blessing. Remember that blessing is nothing else than "to bring bliss" or "to fill something with bliss". Therefore, write something that fills you with bliss about yourself.

Finally, the most important is **C**, the first letter of the word commit. Write down how you are committed to improving your self-esteem. Make a list of the small things you are willing to do to improve how you think and see yourself.

"Life does not happen by chance; it happens by change.".

Dra. Myrelis Aponte Samalot

CHAPTER 4

Strategies for Emotional Homeostasis

When I look back I can see how much I have grown in this area, and also how much I am missing.

As a child, I always liked to participate in everything and was very creative in inventing activities or events among my friends. As I grew up, I was always involved in activities where I took leadership roles. Still in my professional career I have assumed numerous and diverse leadership positions. I have participated in and coordinated events where I have brought together hundreds of people from different parts of the world. When I was young, I didn't realize that being educated in military school made me feel like the boss. That perspective on myself did not allow me to connect with my team. It is only now, years later, that I look back and can understand why so many people saw me that way, as "the boss".

But I learned that I could grow and that my attitude could change. I was able to realize my mistakes and learn how to connect with others.

Here I will share with you some of the strategies that will help you develop a healthy self-esteem, but not only your self-esteem, but your ability to be resilient and to have a healthy and strong emotional intelligence. I assure you that it will help you overcome your adversities.

Educate yourself by reading

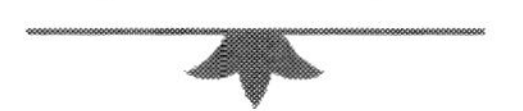

Number one is: educate yourself. Educating yourself doesn't depend on your ability. It's simply a matter of reading for 15 to 30 minutes every day. I know and understand that many women, through no fault of their own, have not had a book in their hands since they were in school. In fact, I know of highly successful people who, without the ability to read, became great entrepreneurs. However, we can all educate ourselves through daily reading.

It is important for us to understand that what we put in our mind programs and plans the way we think and feel. Therefore, if you are planning to strengthen your emotional life, it is crucial that you educate yourself through daily reading.

Listen to me! I know you're busy and sometimes you don't have time for anything else. But I'm sure you can sacrifice 15 to 30 minutes of the time you spend watching TV, on your cell/mobile phone, maybe seeing what others have posted on their social networks. You will notice changes in no time. In fact, you can install on your cell/mobile phone many applications to educate yourself through reading and thus develop your emotional intelligence. This book and guide that you have in your hands, although it is not an application on your cell phone, is an excellent resource to educate yourself.

In fact, my favorite book is the Bible. Many of my business mentors have recommended that I read the Bible. According to them, the Bible is not only extremely ancient, but it is full of teachings that promote or facilitate the development of healthy and strong emotional intelligence. I don't believe I have ever encountered or read a single story in the Bible that does not speak of men and women with healthy self-esteem, a clear self-concept and a godly self-image. Therefore, the Bible can be your best ally. However, I have many authors of books that I like; among them are Napoleon Hill, Camilo Cruz, John C. Maxwell, James Allen and Zig Ziglar.

All of them stand out or are experts on the subject of personal transformation. My friend, reading for me has been key in developing my self-esteem and strengthening my emotional intelligence. If it is not easy for you to dedicate time to reading or you are too lazy to read, follow the recommendations below.

At the beginning, choose only one book. In my case, I have two or three of various subjects around me. I do this because, that way, wherever I am in the house - if I have a minute - I read to fill my brain with information.

Also, always have some kind of bookmark or a system to mark your pages so you know where you left off the last time you read. I fold a tab in the corner of the page where I left off. If both my husband and I are reading the same book, we mark where we left off differently. That way when we read, we each know where we are going in the book.

Another of my recommendations is to join a reading group. One of the best ways to motivate yourself to read is to join a group where everyone is reading the same book, called a mastermind. Typically, the group meets once a week to discuss the content of the book. Group members have a week to read up to a certain point. This "accountability" system promotes what we call a sense of responsibility. In other words, it commits or holds us accountable for reading the assigned pages, and not falling behind. This is good because, although it is not a course, it keeps you actively Reading.

Practice meditation/prayer

The number two strategy to develop emotional intelligence is daily meditation or prayer. Scientific studies show that 10 minutes of daily meditation/prayer strengthens the connection between neurons and keeps frontal lobe areas active.

That is why the Bible teaches us to meditate on His Word every day.

Meditation/prayer provides the necessary time for your brain, or your thoughts, to connect with your spirit and thus strengthen your spiritual self. When you meditate and pray you disconnect from the physical and your intellect, so that you can reach a spiritual sphere or context larger than your reality. Your spiritual life is definitely key to your emotional development.

You may have some myths or false beliefs about what meditation/prayer is. However, meditation/prayer is simply a process of relaxation, where your thinking disconnects from the present and allows you to connect with your inner self, and your Creator.

Meditation/prayer is most effective when practiced during the first few minutes in the morning, as it prepares you for the rest of the day. Meditate for 10 minutes every day to make it part of your daily routine.

Get a Mentor/Coach

The third strategy is to acquire a mentor, in other words, a coach. Identify those people who could be your coach or a role model.

This is the strategy that takes the most work, as not just anyone can, should or qualifies to be your mentor or coach. The person you choose as your mentor must be someone who evidences what they teach and lives what they preach.

You need someone who shows or lives what you are looking for. For example, if you are looking for a mentor in the area of finances, the person must be financially free. A person who is not an expert in managing his or her own finances cannot advise you on how, when or where to invest your money. "It's like preaching morality in your underwear". This phrase very often used on my island describes the above, don't you think?

Your mentor should be someone with whom you have managed to create a relationship whether paid or unpaid, but whose life and example shows the results you are looking for in yours. I'm not talking about your life being like theirs, no. I'm talking about their life modeling your life. I'm talking about their life modeling what you will be inspired to do or develop.

Partner with the right people

The fourth strategy to boost your emotional intelligence to a new level is what kind of people you associate with. Surround yourself with people who have healthy self-esteem, as associating with people with purpose in their lives allows you to grow and move in the same direction.

It is impossible to increase and improve your self-esteem when you are surrounded by people whose self-concept is poor and their self-image is even worse. It does not mean that you give up relationships, perhaps family or friendships, with people who do not have healthy self-esteem. I recommend that you connect with people whose self-esteem is higher than yours and your self-esteem will increase. You will begin to think and talk like people who have healthy self-esteem, people who think positively about themselves.

Positivism

The fifth strategy is to choose the positive side of life. Your brain is able to identify or perceive difficult situations, dangerous events or painful experiences. Fears are the way to escape, as you are innately programmed to run away from any difficult, dangerous or painful situation. However, there is no success to be achieved without having a positive attitude towards what you fear.

Remember that your amygdala and hippocampus react to past experiences. That's why the strategies I mentioned above will help you see the positive side of life. If you choose your mentor well, he or she will help you see the positive side of any situation you find yourself in.

It is also important to stay away from toxic people. You can always identify someone who may be toxic in your life. Toxic people are those who do not believe in you, do not believe in or support your aspirations, are always complaining about something and have a negative perception of life. We all have people like that around us; and, although we should love everyone equally, you have to stay away from people like that. My advice is to limit the time you spend with people who do not bring positive energy into your life.

Finally, stay away from negative information. I started practicing this strategy more than 10 years ago. I learned from one of my business mentors that reading articles, listening on the radio or watching TV shows that are steeped in negativity does nothing positive for my life. So, stay away from all sources of negative information, whether in person or through the media.

Avoid flooding your mind with the results or consequences of catastrophic events, whether local or international. Avoid thoughts that say you can't do what you want to do. Stay away from people who don't have the capacity to think about opportunities.

It is time to look at these tools and, for a moment, analyze which of these strategies you can use to change your way of thinking, improve your quality of life and, therefore, develop your emotional intelligence. Ask yourself which of these strategies you could share with others, because you already use them effectively. So, take a moment to give yourself a chance to assimilate all that I have shared with you. Now answer each of the following questions.

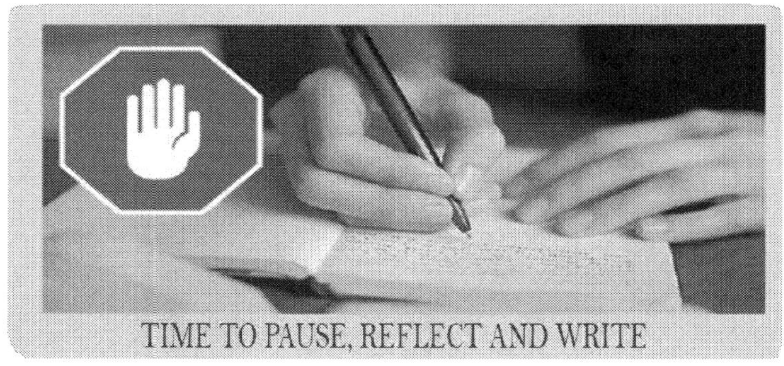

Exercises to develop *Emotional Intelligence*

Education

How much reading time am I achieving per day?
Mark with an **X** or write the time.

_______________ **10 min** ____ **30 min**

_______________ **1 hour** ____ **other**

2. How much reading time can I commit to per day?

_______________ **10 min** ____ **30 min**

_______________ **1 hour** ____ **other**

3. At what time of the day is it easiest for me to read?

   ____in the morning

   ____ at noon

   ____in the afternoon

   ____ in the evening

4. Which book will I start reading as soon as I finish this one?

   ____

   ____

5. What area of my emotional life am I looking to improve with this book?

   ____

   ____

   ____

   ____

   ____

   ____

Meditation/Prayer/Reflection

1. How much meditation, prayer or reflection time am I achieving daily?

   ____

   ____

2. How much time for meditation, prayer or daily reflection can I commit to per day?

   ____

   ____

3. At what time of day do I find it easiest to meditate, pray, or reflect? Why?

____

____

____

____

____

4. What area of my emotional life do I seek to improve with the daily practice of meditation, prayer or reflection?

____

____

____

____

____

____

Mentor *or Coach*

1. How much mentoring or coaching time am I getting per month?

____

____

2. How much mentoring or coaching time can I commit to on a monthly basis?

____

____

3. How can I invest in mentoring or coaching?

____

4. Who can be my mentor or coach?

____

____

____

5. What area of my emotional life am I looking to improve with mentoring or coaching?

____

____

____

____

Association

1. How much time do I spend associating with other positive people?

____

____

2. In what places or groups could you find this support?

____

____

3. What area of my emotional life am I looking to improve with mentoring or coaching?

____

____

Positivism

1. Do I consider myself a positive person?

_____________ **Yes** ____ **No**

2. What things do I do that may seem negative or a complaint?

____

____

____

____

____

____

3. What area of my emotional life do I seek to improve by being more positive?

____

____

____

____

____

____

3

PART

SHARE YOUR TALENTS

"I alone cannot change the world but I can throw a stone across the water to create many ripples".

'Every work of love, carried out wholeheartedly, will always succeed in bringing people closer to God.".

Mother Teresa of Calcutta

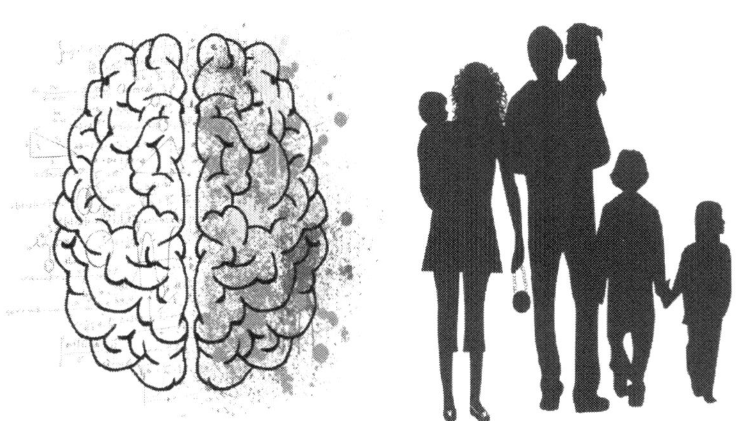

= environment / society / family

CHAPTER 5

Your Social Intelligence

The roles of women

I still remember the day I found out I was pregnant with my first daughter, Victoria. Being an only child and growing up alone with my mother, I only had role models in my aunts or closest relatives. As I grew up, although as a child I dreamed of getting married and having children, over time those dreams transformed. Getting married and having children were no longer a priority. I had become so dedicated to my career and the community that I had forgotten that I could form my own community: my family.

My husband, on the other hand, came from a family of four siblings and many nieces and nephews, so he dreamed of a family like his siblings. Needless to say, how much joy everyone in the family felt, especially the future grandparents. But, to be honest - my dear friend - deep down I was surprised and somewhat terrified. In this process I discovered that pregnancy ended up being the most beautiful stage of my life. I miss every moment, the positive anxiety of waiting and the role that from birth onwards would entail.

Actually, no one prepares us for such changes, physically, emotionally and socially. I remember people who could not believe I was pregnant. They could not visualize me as a mother, as I loved my career and was fascinated by traveling. Honestly, housework has never been a favorite of mine.

But the arrival of my daughter Victoria represented one of the most impactful moments of my life. She has been the ***catalyst*** that propelled the improvement of my quality of life. Valeria, my second daughter, gave me the opportunity to experience new stages and face challenges that have also strengthened my life.

I've had people ask me: Don't you miss the single life? In all honesty, I had a lot of choices, freedom, and less worries, but I didn't really live. Being a mother allowed me to experience unconditional love. So, as complicated as my life may seem caring for two young lives, I don't want to go back. The key to success as a wife, mother, and a professional lies in a balanced life or a state of family *homeostasis*. The continuous search for balance in my family life has been a path of exploration and learning.

The family, or the nuclear family, is the basis of all society. Without family there is simply no society. On the other hand, the society to which we belong allows us to live lives filled with experiences involving members of our community. These experiences have immense power. They influence the way we think and act. The environment that surrounds us sometimes determines the decisions we make on a daily basis. It impacts our family life and the roles we assume in society.

Did you know that we have the ability to change our environment or our surroundings? In fact, the frontal lobe in the cerebral cortex has areas that interpret social interaction. If you look at the image, you will see that in the frontal lobe, there is an area called Broca, where precisely our linguistic and oral skills originate. It is there where -in addition- behavior, attention, planning and other cognitive skills that allow us to socialize are managed.

Social and interpersonal intelligence is found in this brain area. This type of intelligence or capacity is part of the multiple intelligences that I have shared with you previously. In this case, social intelligence is defined as the ability to feel empathy or the ability to relate well with others. In the world that you and I live in, we are surrounded by people. Without people, there would be no world, right? Therefore, our social intelligence includes our ability to relate and adjust to social, generational and global changes.

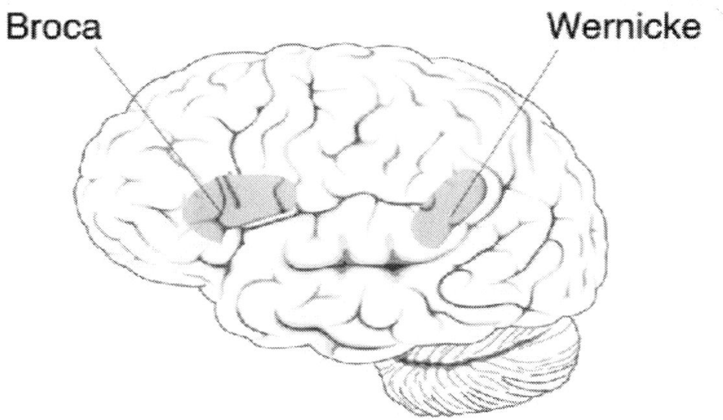

According to technology and media, we have had to expand all these abilities. The world is accessible at the touch of a button on our cell/mobile phone and this changes from one moment to the next. The role of communications has been beneficial, but it has also affected our family, professional, and community roles.

At a time when we have experienced a global pandemic that has specifically marked the way we connect as a society, this topic becomes even more relevant. This global event has made us find new ways to relate to each other and stay connected, even in the midst of a necessary physical-social distancing. Therefore, developing and strengthening your social and interpersonal interaction skills will serve as useful tools as you move into decades of new challenges. I want to talk to you about various roles, before understanding a little more about how to improve our social intelligence.

The Family Role

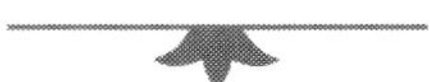

As a Latina woman we have a very strong family role in our culture. We can be very attached to your loved ones. This may include: your parents, spouse and children, siblings, grandparents, cousins, among others. In fact, as a woman, wife and mother, the culture assumes a high position of leadership. You may already be experiencing or assuming the matriarchal role that brings with it the administrative responsibility for the home and family. The matriarchal role is essential and intensely important. You are a wife, mother, daughter, sister, aunt, cousin, granddaughter, among many other possible roles within your family.

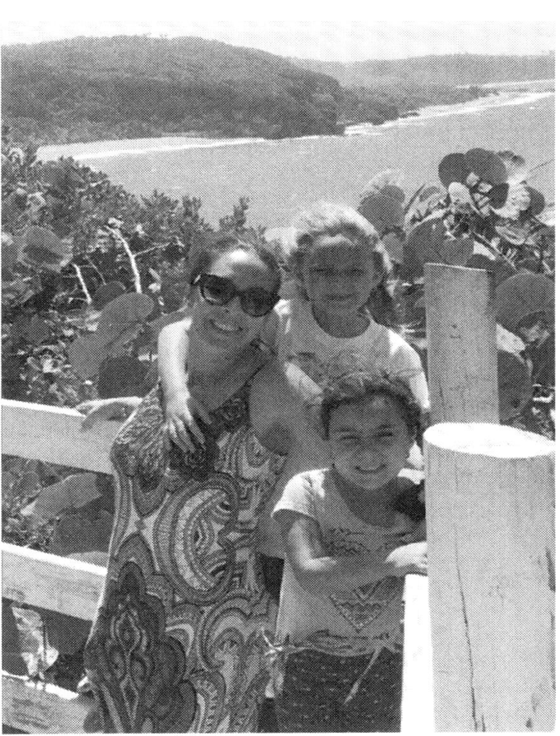

The role you play within your family is extremely complex and takes up a large part of your daily schedule. Being a wife, mother, daughter, among others, can be complicated, take up a lot of your time, impact your health and demand a lot of emotional intelligence. Your roles within the family entail emotional responsibilities with each of your loved ones.

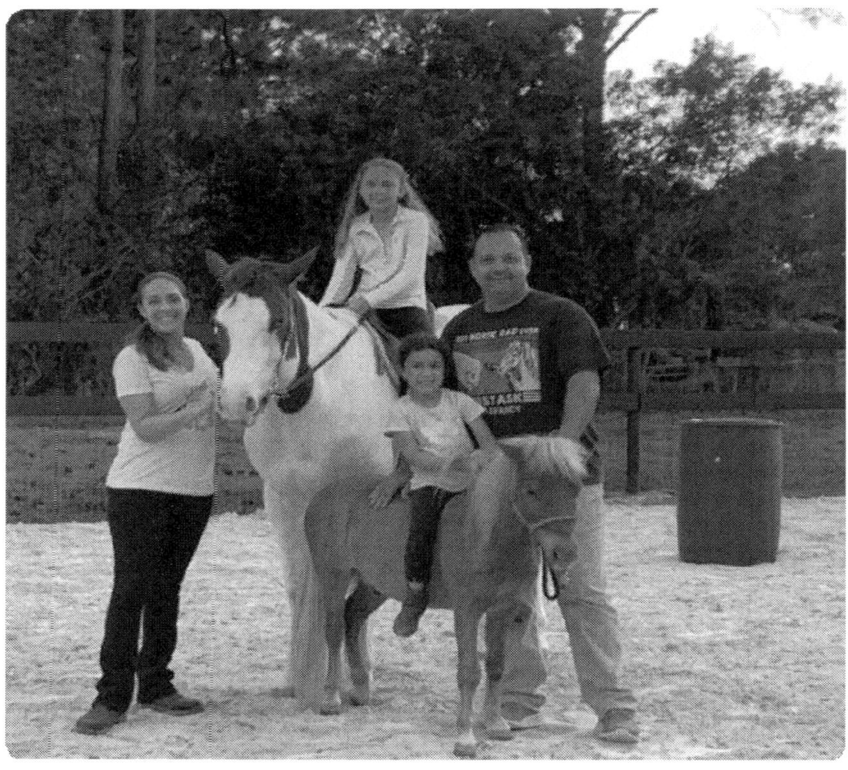

In fact, this family role responds to the most important stages of Maslow's Pyramid that I mentioned in the introduction of this book. It is up to you to make your family members feel secure, accepted and loved. Therefore, this family role brings with it a number of complexities and challenges that you must overcome. Take a minute to analyze and answer the following questions:

- What role(s) do I have as a member of my family?
- What strength am I bringing to my family?
- What problems or situations have I brought to the nuclear family?
- Am I the link that binds my family together or the one that breaks it?

These are questions you should ask yourself, but not to judge yourself. Never! As you have seen in the previous chapters, this also has a solution. Remember that the many responsibilities within your family can be affected by a lack of emotional intelligence. But we will make this better!

Location in the world

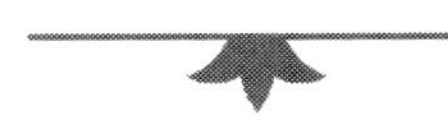

Women generally want to fulfill all of our roles efficiently and effectively. I think it is important
for you to take some time to understand where you fit in the world. What do I mean by fit? Your place in the world depends on how clear you are about your roles, what roles you accept, what roles you reject, and how they are impacted by your beliefs.

Your belief system decrees who you are and how you behave. These beliefs have been determined or influenced by your experiences since childhood. For example, how do you remember your mother? What example did she set for you? Was your mother happy or long-suffering?

Was your mother loving or did she never express affection? Was your mother industrious or listless? Was your mother respected and admired or abused and despised? All of your experiences as a child have created your belief system. They are stored in your unconscious and long-term memory. Bringing this to your awareness will help you better understand your role in the world and what you can contribute to your transformation process. I should add that your location in the world has also been influenced by the role men have played in your life. Was your father present or absent in your life?

Was your father affectionate or dry with you? Was your father hardworking and a good provider or lazy and a poor provider? Likewise, the experiences you have had with grandfathers, uncles or an ex-spouse have influenced the beliefs that dictate your roles in the world. Negative experiences with men in your life, whether in the past or present, have created a false and pervasive belief system that is carried throughout your life. Therefore, it is imperative that you bring those experiences in your unconscious to the conscious level.

These experiences, however diverse they may be, create patterns or mental repetitions that make our brain create conclusions about what we have experienced. We see women who cannot trust a man because, at some point, a man was unfaithful. We can see women who even abuse their husbands because they lived experiences where they learned to protect themselves from men. These examples, although very generic, help us understand how previous experiences create a belief system that determines how, when and where we are going to act.

My recommendation is that you continue with an exploratory attitude and, above all, don't judge yourself. You have come this far in reading this book. You have already been able to recognize and understand the areas where you need to grow in order to live a life full of health and stability. Now, you need to focus! Focus on working to strengthen your emotional intelligence in an intentional way. This will help you better understand your place in the world. In this way you will be even better able to generate a social environment that allows you to create, develop and strengthen relationships within your family and in whatever social setting you are in.

Finally, your location in the world will be determined or influenced by the roles you have played in society. influenced by the roles or roles you have played in society.

What role have you taken in society; how did you learn to interact with others? As I explained earlier, your belief system impacts every scenario you encounter in life.

Many women reach adulthood without understanding what they are in this world for. Sad, isn't it? They have not found purpose and feel lost at times. This lack of purpose and derailment is not caused by a lack of intelligence, skills or abilities; it is caused by a lack of awareness of who we are and what we can contribute.

We are beings of social interaction. We are created to relate and we can choose with whom. But this will depend on your belief system. Ultimately, it is your beliefs that will determine whether you will achieve the social success you crave in life.

In your hands lies the course of your social success! In the next few lines, I will talk a little more about this.

Moral values

Moral values are defined as a set of norms and customs that are transmitted by society to everyone. They also represent the good or correct way to act or behave in any social environment we find ourselves in. They allow us to differentiate between good and bad, right and wrong, just and unfair.

Moral values are introduced from childhood by our parents or authority figures. Then, in school, they are reinforced by teachers or professors. Many of our moral values are acquired through the religion we practice. Other values are associated with the society to which we belong and violating them can even lead to legal sanctions. Some moral values are: honesty, respect, gratitude, loyalty, tolerance, solidarity, generosity, friendship, kindness and humility, among others.

We can also see hierarchical scales among moral values. For example, in the midst of a conflict, we may be forced to choose or decide between values. For example, loyalty is fundamental in a friendship.

However, if a friend has committed a crime and we are questioned by the police, the right thing to do would be to privilege the value of honesty over our loyalty. In conclusion, moral values are essential to achieve an atmosphere of harmony and coexistence in society.

Ethical values

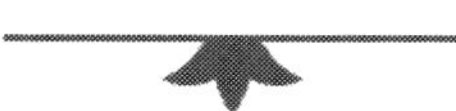

Although many people think that moral and ethical values are the same, it is important to see that there is a great difference between them. Ethical values are created by a series of norms or rules that regulate the conduct of individuals, such as truth, justice, freedom and responsibility. Moral values, on the other hand, as I said before, refer to the set of common practices or customs of a society, and are aimed at establishing a differentiation between the correct or positive way of acting, and the incorrect or negative way of acting.

Etymologically, the word ethics originates from the Greek word *estos*, which means "habit or custom". Therefore, ethical values are behavioral guidelines that regulate a person's conduct. First of all, ethics is a branch of philosophy that studies what is moral and performs an analysis of the moral system to be applied at the individual and social level. Among the most relevant ethical values are: justice, freedom, respect, responsibility, integrity, loyalty, honesty, equity, among others.

You acquire ethical values during your individual development, through experiences in your family, social and school environment, or even through the media. Ethical values demonstrate your personality. In other words, your conduct or the way you behave will create a positive or negative image of yourself. Ethical values can be seen through your convictions, feelings and interests.

For example, a person who fights for justice and freedom of human beings reflects a just person and therefore has a positive image.

A person who is against human rights and supports injustice is perceived as an apathetic person and as a result has a negative image. Therefore, ethical values allow to regulate behavior, to achieve collective welfare, and a harmonious and peaceful coexistence in society.

Take into consideration the importance of understanding your place in the world. Pay close attention to the influence that moral and ethical values have on your daily life as a member of society. You can see that the role you play, inside and outside the family, is of utmost importance and great influence in the world we live in. Knowing yourself will be key to your social development.

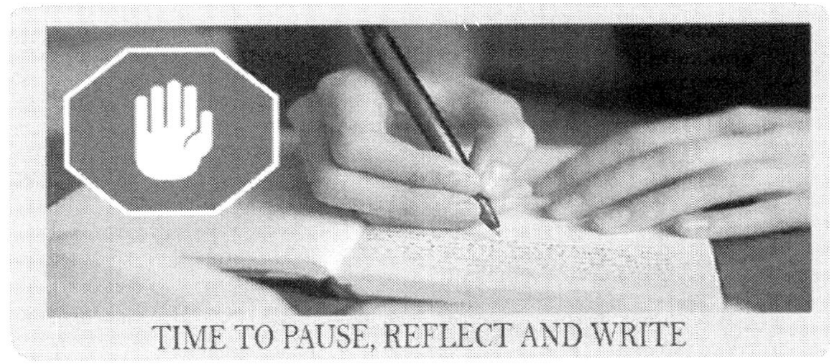

Exercises to develop *Social Intelligence*

Now, to begin to work on yourself, answer some of these questions. Do not look for perfect answers; now you are going to express in your own words whatever comes to your awareness. This will help you define yourself. Remember, do not judge your thoughts.

1. How do I define who I am in my family role?

____

____

____

____

____

2. How do I contribute to my social environments?

____

____

____

____

3. What moral values are important to me?
   to me? Define them in your own words

____

____

____

____

4. What ethical values are most important to me? Define them in your own words

____

____

____

____

Professional role

Now, when we add our professional role, everything starts to intertwine. As women, we have definitely faced and continue to face all kinds of challenges. You may have studied in your home country, pursued a career and achieved a certain level of professional success. Being away from your country, you feel that all your academic and professional achievements are gone, and you no longer know what to do. Likewise, you may not have a college degree, but you have a number of talents and skills that include visual, manual and culinary arts. You know you have so many strengths and great potential; but you find yourself without direction. You don't know where to start.

You may be growing in your job, but your family roles are being affected. You may be having a very rewarding family role; but you are feeling that you are not progressing in your professional role.

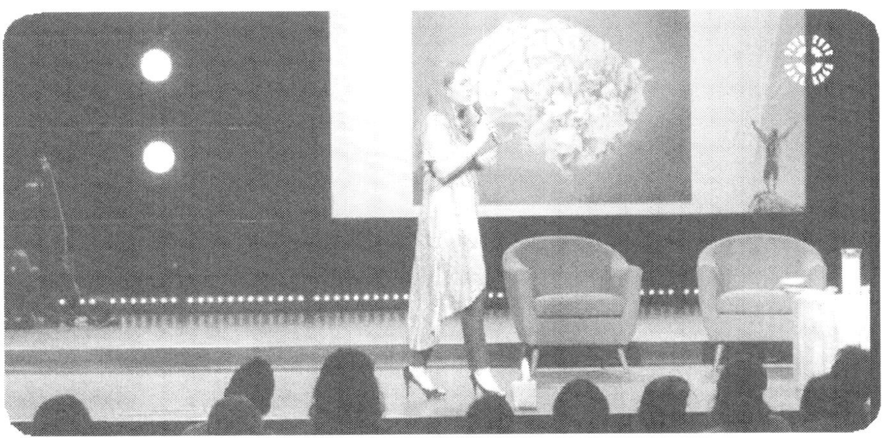

Both you and I know that the professional role is the gateway to income-generating opportunities that benefit the entire family. On the other hand, your professional role can be the precursor to high levels of stress, due to the long hours or intense work involved in your career. In addition, it can make you feel physically exhausted and unfocused.

We must also recognize that all professional roles around the world are changing exponentially. We have to prepare ourselves to be ready for the changes. They alter our balance; and it is for that, and many other reasons, that we need to develop our emotional intelligence.

Emotional intelligence plays an important role in the development of our family and professional role. You may have arrived in the United States and suddenly feel that all your talents are not being utilized as you want and expect. You may not be proficient in English and your lack of proficiency in the language has become a stumbling block that prevents you from capitalizing on your skills. You have made countless efforts with few results. Time passes and you are not where you want to be. But my friend, I have something to tell you: Stop! Stop harboring negative thoughts.

At this point, you must develop your social intelligence using your emotional intelligence in order to move forward. Let me share with you a great truth. 80% of the times we don't achieve what we want is due to a negative attitude towards what we are trying to achieve. Only 20% is due to lack of knowledge or skills. In other words, attitude precedes or is more important than skill.

Our family and professional roles come together to enable us to make a difference in the world we live in. In reality, we are citizens of the world and therefore have to contribute to the good of humanity. How do you discover this? I'll explain in this next section.

Purpose

Sometimes, we have developed a professional life that is not connected to our purpose. It could be that your career is not connected to what you are truly passionate about, your talents and skills. Did you know that 60% of working people are dissatisfied with their careers? 75% of employees, or people on track in their various careers, would like to start over, but lack the motivation to take the plunge. They want something new for their lives, but lack, as they say in my country, "the will to do it". This lack of motivation or desire may be because they don't know what their purpose in life is. Within the context of this book and guide, purpose means:

1. A firm determination to do something. For example, "I have decided to learn English to get ahead in this country", or "I am going to orient myself to start a new business".
2. Having a clear objective of what you want to achieve. For example, "The purpose of this book is to raise the consciousness of woman, so that they can reach their highest potential and find personal and professional homeostasis.

The best vehicle for finding your purpose in life is reflection, and this takes time. If you are a woman of faith, reflection plays an important role in your life. Why? Because a woman who is fervent in her faith, or who cultivates her spiritual life, knows that reflection will help her understand what she was created to do and what her mission in life is.

When you were little, someone may have told you, "Go to school and get a degree so you can get a good job later". Maybe you didn't get a career, but you learned numerous skills that enable you to work and support yourself. However, I assure you that no one asked you: What is your purpose in life or what is your passion or what do you dream of achieving in life?

Did you know that most people identify or define themselves by their profession? The first question we typically ask is, "What do you do for a living?" We all answer, "I'm a teacher," "I'm an engineer," or "I'm a doctor." They think or feel that profession dictates their purpose in life. However, purpose in a person's life goes beyond pleasure or passion. Purpose gives you meaning and purpose in life.

When you find your meaning in life, your whole being comes into **harmony**. *Harmony* is one of my favorite words because *harmony* is defined as balance. It is the proportion and proper correspondence between the different elements of a whole. *Harmony* is also defined as peace, concord and understanding between two or more people. Therefore, at this point I can conclude that *homeostasis* equals balance and balance needs *harmony*.

When you find your purpose all your roles in life will begin to coincide. Like a good jigsaw puzzle, each piece of your life will fall into its right place. Little by little, by putting each piece in its place, the time will come when you will be able to have the complete vision of what your life will look like. I assure you that as you find purpose and *harmony*, you will find balance in all phases of your life. Be patient! As your picture becomes clearer you will be able to see and find the missing pieces.

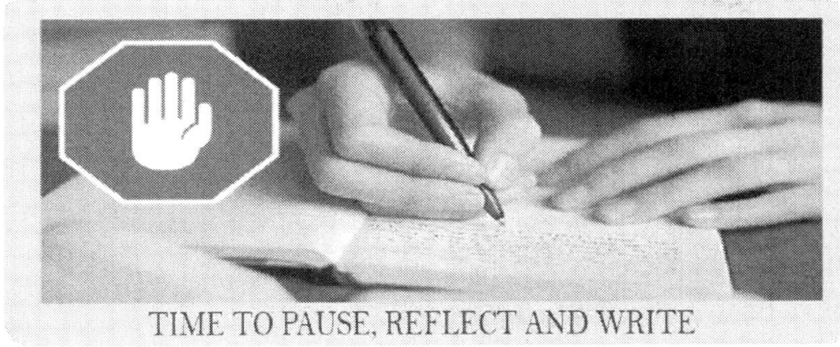

Exercises to develop *Social Intelligence*

Finding your purpose will be a great exercise in introspection. How can you get started? Write down the answers to the following questions.

1. Today, what has brought purpose to my life?

____

____

____

____

2. Which things give me pleasure?

____

____

____

____

3. What passion do I have that makes me feel full of life?

____

____

____

____

4. How is this passion part of my purpose?

____

____

____

____

5. Is my current career or profession related to my purpose, how?

____

____

____

____

6. If what I am currently doing does not connect me to my purpose, what can I do to move in the direction of my purpose in life?

____

____

____

____

These questions are not designed to make you feel frustrated that you are not in the right place. On the contrary, the idea is that today is your first step to a life full of purpose and harmony. In that way, you will find homeostasis or balance in your career.

Progress

Once you understand what your purpose in life is, the steps to take -or how to progress toward that purpose- will come to mind almost automatically. What does it mean to progress? Progress or making progress is the end result of continuous activities, or actions, in the direction of your purpose. In other words, once you find your purpose you can then design and establish a plan of action.

There is no progress without strategies for dealing with change. The world around you and the culture of this country are continually changing. Technology has caused us to be constantly accelerating. Our transformation process is essential to adjust and be in constant harmony, not only with all these changes, but also with the continuous rush. On the one hand, change and speed will open doors to new opportunities to progress and achieve your purpose in life. On the other hand, resistance to change and fast-paced life will not allow you to progress.

You will be able to move from where you are to a position of progress if you are willing to see the world in a different way than you may have learned from your parents, family and culture. I don't mean abandoning your ethical values, morals and much less your faith. On the road to progress, these three pieces are essential to keep you centered in who you are. Now, flexibility and a willingness to learn new things quickly will be your career companions. Once you have found your purpose and are on the road to advancement, your ability to move with the changes will be one of the keys to your professional success.

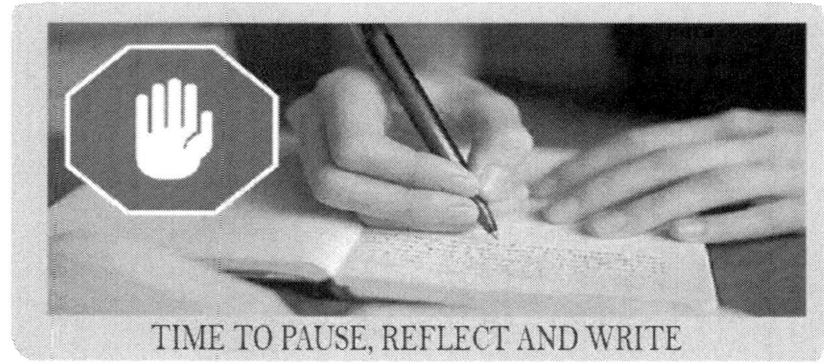

Exercises to develop *Social Intelligence*

Action plan

I think you are now ready to develop your first action plan. As in the previous exercises, now answer the following question. Your answer will help you organize your thoughts to help your plans become clearer and take the shape that leads to your professional success.

What are the three goals you would like to achieve in the next 12 months?

Goal 1:______________________________________

Goal 2:______________________________________

Goal 3:______________________________________

Community role

Your Talents or skills

It is important to see where your talents can contribute to the community. When we contribute positively, our passions are discovered.

Our brain begins to create new connections and neurochemicals of pleasure and well-being are released. As a result of helping others, your physical and emotional health improves, which will lead to complete *homeostasis.*In addition, service brings a sense of belonging and purpose in life.

What talents do you have to offer, and how can you use the skills you enjoy most to improve?

the quality of life for others? Your social or community role should be based on the impact and influence you can have on others, whether in your home, the place where you work, or in your community.

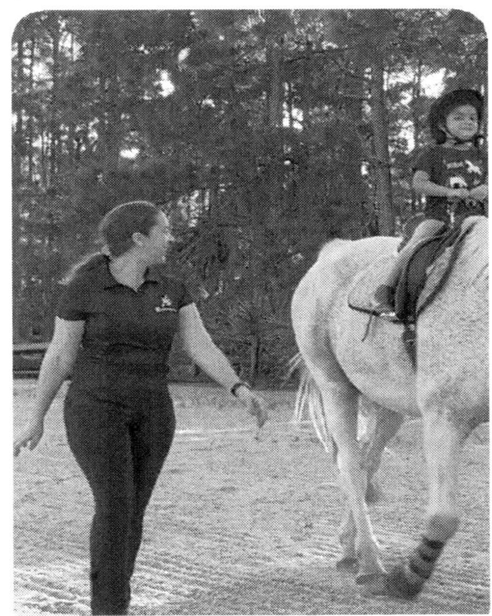

Personally, I love to offer others joy, hope and opportunities to thrive. I also ask myself, what am I leaving my daughters? Have you ever thought about this? I ask myself this question every day. My husband - sometimes- looks at me in amazement and asks, "Are you considering doing anything else for the girls? And I reply, "Whether I go overboard or not, I don't know. But I do know that I enjoy it!"

For example, my oldest girl, Victoria, was only 4 years old when she started competing riding Puerto Rican Paso Fino horses. I rode when I was little. I always loved horses and enjoyed it casually. But, when she started competing, I was invited to train and participate in some riding competitions.

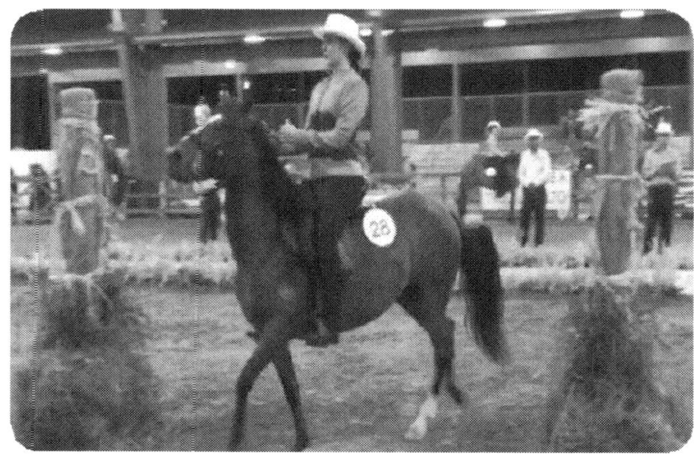

While I had many friends who told me it would be beautiful, there were others who told me I was daring to compete with women who had more than 20 years of experience. However, when I realized the level of influence and impact it would have on my daughter, I took the courage to take on the challenge. You know what? Although I didn't win any awards, I was eliminated along with many of those with 20 years of experience. So, it was worth it! Along the way I rediscovered a passion that I now enjoy with my daughter, my family and many others.

"Our spirit is the author of our intellect and the protector of our body."

Dra. Myrelis Aponte Samalot

Service

I want you to ask yourself today where and how you can contribute to your community. This will make your roles take on deep meaning. Serving others is essential for us to find purpose in our lives. Even if you are already progressing in your professional life, service to others or your community role will take you to a higher and more encompassing level. In fact, the pleasure that serving brings an even greater sense of peace, *harmony* and balance than career advancement.

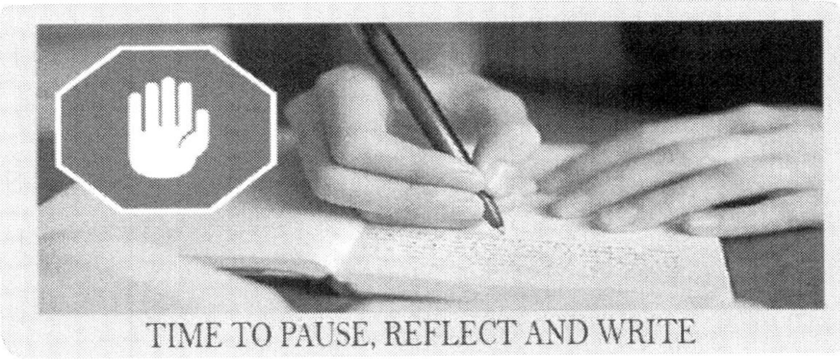

Exercises to develop *Social Intelligence*
Mi Mark

I would like at this time to trace your dominant hand. This exercise is very interesting, as it will activate your thinking zones.

Then, answer the questions next to each finger. This exercise allows introspection.

- Where am I?
- Where do I help?
- Where am I going?

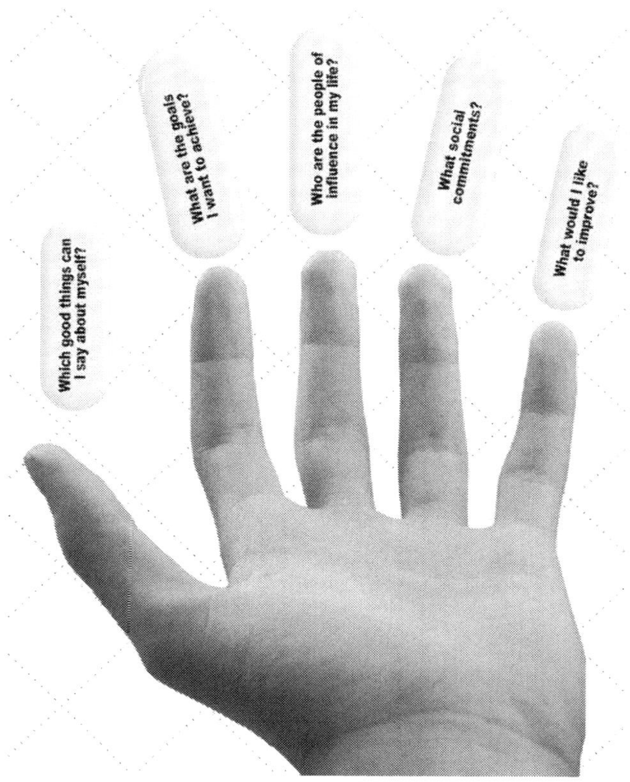

Now trace your dominant hand

The Influence

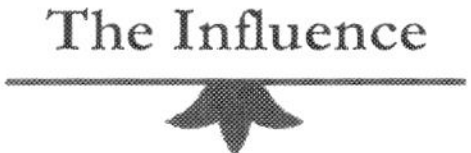

As active members of a community, we all possess the ability to have a high level of influence on those around us. Consciously or unconsciously, your influences are your children, partner, family, co-workers and those you serve.

There is a lot of power in influence. In fact, it happens most of the time indirectly. There are people whose purpose is to influence the lives of people they don't even know. For example, the primary job of the media, including social media, is to influence the lives of the people they reach. Take a good look. When you watch any TV show or listen to the radio, you are bombarded with commercials that want to convince you to buy some product, vote for some person or contribute financially to some cause. In one way or another, they will influence your life from what you eat, how you dress or who you vote for, among many other things. Influence is defined by experts in human behavior as the power of a person, or thing, to determine or alter the way another person thinks or acts. It is also defined as, the effect, consequence or change produced by one thing or person on another person.

How powerful influence is! It is important that we recognize that you, in every role you play in life, have the strength or power to change the way people within your sphere of influence think or act. Now, the key or the secret is that you accept that you have the power to influence others and understand how you can do it. Without even thinking about it, the way you think, make decisions and act makes you a powerful influencer on a daily basis.

Awareness of our power to influence others is the key to impacting our families, our colleagues and, ultimately, our community. However, in order to influence others, I must assume or achieve a position of leadership. So, let's explore some keys to leadership.

Leadership

I have had the privilege of being mentored by leaders of international stature such as John C. Maxwell, Paul Martinelli, Roddy Galbraith, Pedro and Patricia Lizardi, Eduardo Perez, Ivan and Carmen Morales, Mario Orzini, Dr. Carmen Inoa Vazquez and Dr. Lourdes Allen, to name a few. Each of these leaders demonstrate characteristics that empower them to positively impact the people they encounter in their life's journey.

First, each of these leaders demonstrates the ability to believe. Whenever I personally interact with them, I can see that they believe what they want to achieve, they can achieve it. There is no doubt in them that they can achieve what they set out to do. When you listen to their stories you realize, just like any other human being, that there were moments of total difficulty in their lives. However, if there is one thing they never practiced, nor do they practice, it is a lack of belief or faith in achieving their dreams.

These leaders not only believe, but they transfer that ability to believe in others. It is as if believing is a seed that they sow in the people around them. True leaders help us to see the many opportunities that today's changing world offers us. Through this book and guide I want to sow in your heart the same seed of belief that these leaders have sown and cultivated in my life.

Stop and think for a moment about who is currently sowing and cultivating in your life the ability to believe in your potential for progress. In addition, I want you to think about those people who have sown the seed of faith. Who are you helping to believe? Who or whom are you instilling faith in? Instilling faith in others will strengthen your own faith and lead to self-realization, *harmony* and balance.

The second thing I've noticed about people who excel in leadership-or those who have influenced my life-is that they don't use intimidation and fear to get their followers to follow themTrue leaders use their influential energy to model the lifestyle that is achievable. In other words, a true leader is charismatic. Their captivating energy and focus are unaffected by circumstances, as they believe in their goal and have the faith to achieve it regardless of the circumstances.

During this pandemic caused by COVID-19, I have been able to see in them that, despite the great challenges they face, they do not lose faith or charisma. On the contrary, what I admire is that I see them more determined than ever to achieve purpose in their lives. A true leader is consistent and does not stop in the face of circumstances. This does not mean that they are not capable of experiencing uncertainty, frustration and a lot of pain. What it does mean is that their faith lifts them up and moves them beyond the circumstances. Sharing their energy with others is what allows them to keep moving in the right direction. You know what I've seen happen with their companies, programs and projects, that in times of uncertainty their creativity is unleashed, and instead of falling behind, they achieve unprecedented victories.

So, for a moment, think about your grace and energy - are you charismatic, can you positively influence others? You may feel that your energy level is not optimal. See if, when you talk to others, you transmit your positive energy and your faith, in other words, your charisma, because after all, this will set you apart from others. Like a magnet you will attract people and be a blessing to others. Your level of charisma impacts your level of influence.

The third characteristic of these leaders is the way they are committed. They take their responsibilities extremely seriously. They are committed not only to their projects, organizations or companies, but also to all the people they serve. In the midst of difficult times, they never back down, but accelerate to meet their commitments.

Leaders commit to doing something when they believe they must do it and believe they have the ability to do it. Therefore, leaders' belief drives them to action. How we commit ourselves shows what our priorities are. The way you serve others, the quality of your service and your consistency regardless of whether or not you have personal gains, makes others identify this characteristic in you. The quality of your commitment determines your level of influence.

There are people who want to be in a leadership role, but are the last to arrive and the first to leave. These are people who are unwilling to commit. They don't put in the time and effort necessary for what needs to be accomplished to be accomplished. True leaders are distinguished because they are the first to arrive and the last to leave. They do whatever they have to do to get the desired results.

If you want to be a person of influence and bring about positive change in the lives of others, you must believe, exhibit charisma and be committed. These three characteristics are essential for you to be an effective leader. If you lack or are low in any of these characteristics, don't be discouraged. Now that you are aware of the essential characteristics of a leader, I know you will put into practice strategies that will help you develop your leadership role.

Legacy

The last thing in the discussion about our communal or social role is legacy. We have talked about your talents or abilities, the importance of serving humanity, the influence you have on others, and your ability to lead or exercise leadership positions.

Legacy or the blessing of leaving a legacy goes far beyond what we have talked about. Very few people think about this until they are already in their beautiful sunset. One of the main reasons we don't think about our legacy is because we spend half our lives without having found our purpose. However, once we find it, leaving a legacy becomes relevant.

Many people think that a legacy is only what I leave to my family. In fact, by definition, a legacy means a material or immaterial thing that is left in a will or passed on from parents to children, from generation to generation. But, if we are considering that we are citizens of the world, then my legacy goes beyond my family environment.

We don't know how long we are on this earth, but if we live with purpose, every minute counts. When we are saying goodbye to a loved one, we always hear people describe the best things about the person who left. What did we learn from that person, how did that person inspire us, how did that person help us face challenges in life? We know that no matter how troubled that person was, at the time of their death there will always be people who loved them in life and speak positively about what they left behind, whether it was their smile, their jokes, or their way of doing things. I think that all of us, when we leave this world, always leave something behind, whether material or immaterial.

Today, I want you to think about what you want to leave behind. What positive influence do you want to leave in your family, in your profession or in your community? At a very young age, I had the opportunity to learn sign language in Puerto Rico.

I started learning from a group of deaf people in the church I attended. Such was my interest that in addition to learning songs, I used all the resources available to me to become proficient. I improved my skills and by the age of 19 I was already providing professional interpreting services. Those were years of much growth.

I was studying Natural Sciences in college at the time. As the years went by, I decided to pursue a Master's degree in Counseling with a specialty in Deafness.

However, at that time, the problem of interpreter training in Puerto Rico was limited and did not meet the needs of the Deaf community.

I got to the point of getting involved in professional organizations in Puerto Rico and in the United States to contribute to legislative processes that would benefit the Deaf community in Puerto Rico. It was there that I began to teach other interested people sign language. What was my goal? To offer quality services to the deaf population in my country.

In 2005, as I was finishing my last year of doctoral studies in Puerto Rico, together with another great colleague I began to create the first university level academic program for Sign Language Interpreters in Puerto Rico. The Ana G. Méndez University System shared the vision and gave me the space to create a bachelor's degree program. You see? It was there that my opportunity to leave a legacy in the interpreting profession in Puerto Rico began.

In January 2006, the program began. I managed to get scholarships to students and see four groups graduate before taking the next step in my career. Today I live with the pride that this program still exists, thanks to the fact that one day I accepted the challenge and believed it was possible. You must believe it! Although I never received recognition for what I did, I got the best gift of all. I was the precursor or *catalyst* of the university program that trains and empowers those who want to serve the Deaf community in Puerto Rico.

I still have many legacies to fulfill at the family, professional and community levels. These play a very important role in my purpose in life. I'm sure you've made some legacies for your generation. But if you still feel you haven't and are discovering your purpose, now is your time.

Whether you are a mother, grandmother or aunt, I believe one of the most valuable and purposeful roles is to educate our next generation. I remind you that we are citizens of the world. If you have been reading this book and guide it is because you desire a balanced life for yourself and safely for those around you. Serving the community by educating the next generation will make you part of a cause greater than yourself.

Our children and youth need role models that will allow them to see a bright and worthwhile future. At times, we see them turn away from their parents, grandparents and aunts and uncles because they see brighter role models outside their family environment. So, let's provide an environment of possibility that shines brighter than the external noise. To do that, you need to put into practice the same characteristics of the leaders I spoke about earlier. You must believe in your abilities, positively influence people within your sphere of influence and, above all, be committed to serving those who can benefit from your gifts.

To conclude this chapter on your communal or social role, I want to tell you that with children and young people it will be necessary for you to demonstrate a high degree of belief or faith, not only in them, but in yourself. This new generation has the ability to see when we are not sincere. We have to believe in them until they learn to believe in themselves. Talk to them about their possibilities. Don't limit where they will go, because remember that they may be here for much longer than you and, therefore, you will not be able to see the end of their story.

Share your charisma. Share the energy to live and serve. Technology has brought the world closer together, but it has pushed people apart in many ways. Find ways to connect with others. In this pandemic time let the young people in your family see you survive and flourish by making use of technology. Let them see you not only work from home, but also monitor their virtual education and stay connected to others.

Commit to being a mentor to your next generation. Identify a young woman, girl or group that you can serve. Do it with the purpose of leaving a legacy of hope in others. It doesn't matter in what area you serve, but serve and leave a piece of yourself in your youth. Leaving a legacy is the segment in your life that will make you invincible and unbreakable. You will feel harmony and your being will feel a homeostasis and balance beyond measure.

C HAPTER

6

Strategies to find your Social Homeostasis

Identify your purpose. What is your calling?

As we have discussed in the previous chapters, we can achieve social equilibrium. But this balance or *homeostasis* is only achieved when we understand who we are and what our purpose in life is. Who are you? What is your calling in life? If you know who you are and what your purpose in life is, then you will know what you are going to contribute and how you are going to do it.

This could be difficult as it happened to me, I had several talents and I didn't focus on just one. I wanted to do more than I could. It was difficult because I only had the discipline to maintain and develop one at a time. Having many talents seems wonderful, but in reality, it is challenging and stressful. Because you can't reach your full potential in several areas at once.

There is a saying in Puerto Rico that goes, "El que mucho abarca, poco aprieta"(Jack of all trades, master of none). It wasn't until I had the opportunity to become a mother that I found that my primary purpose in life was to share my own experiences of growth with many, many people including you.

I learned that sharing with others what I have learned on my journey towards *homeostasis* was the best way to help those who yearn for balance and *harmony* in their lives.

Identify your priorities What is most important to you?

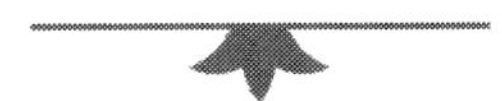

I had to believe that my dreams would come true. Nothing is impossible for those who believe. My motherhood did not mean not being me. In order to make my dreams come true, I had to take the necessary steps to fulfill all the various roles in my life.

Women face numerous challenges on a daily basis - they are incalculable! We have to take care of the children, the husband or partner and the house. As if that weren't enough, many of us also have careers or trades that demand our attention. However, when we are determined to be successful at everything, we look for ways to fulfill our responsibilities without falling into madness. We seek to assume our roles in a balanced way.

Personally, for me it was extremely important to discover that my priority was my family; that everything I do is for them, with them and for them; that it fills me with pleasure and joy to give the best of myself in order to be, to do and to have. Being successful is not a sinful word. Rather, it is a word that drives us to achieve our full potential in life.

Achieving social balance will depend on what your priorities are. Once you understand or have determined what your priorities are, you will be able to find and implement the strategies to achieve your social goals or fulfill your community role.

One strategy that could be incredibly effective for you - and could also create family bonding - is the creation of a Dream and Goal Board. This is a space in your home where you creatively display what you long to achieve in life that includes your yearnings and goals you want to accomplish. In this area you can also include the dreams and goals of each of your family members. Why not?

Take a space on one of the walls of your home where everyone can see

the Dream Board every day. Cut out pictures and place them on a poster that you will put in this space. Write dates by which you and your family want to achieve those goals and dreams. Review and visit the poster daily. This helps everyone in the household collaborate and stay focused.

The Dream Board will help you focus on your priorities so you don't get distracted by activities that don't enrich you or lead you to your purpose. This strategy keeps everyone in the household on track with their goals. It helps your children focus on their future and the experiences they want to have. The Dream Board is a no-holds-barred strategy.

For example, we included pictures of our two daughters' births. Rather, my husband posted them. The girls, on the other hand, cut out a picture of a playhouse for the backyard from a magazine. They colored this image on the Dream Board to indicate the dream of someday being able to play inside that playhouse, in the backyard. The dream came true! We all also put the picture of a house where we could have horses. Today, as I finish this book, that dream also came true. Try it, at first it will seem odd, but once you do the first you will love to continue to build on it I promise!

Maintain communication in your family

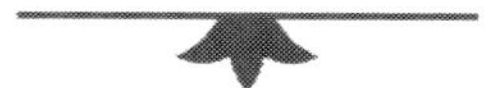

I also recommend that you share your priorities with your nuclear family. I don't think we should be feminists, but socialists. To achieve *homeostasis* within our social role we have to clearly communicate our priorities, desires and dreams with the people we live with. That way you can also live a balanced family life. The secret is to communicate clearly.

Communicate what are the expectations of each of the members of your household, your nuclear family. When you have created your own family, your priorities are your marriage and children. Therefore, get involved in what concerns your partner and children.

What I am about to say may be controversial. If you have a healthy relationship with your children, your spouse should be your first priority, not the children. And that is, of course, if your husband is the father of your children. Now, if you have remarried, the home situation may be different, especially when you live with children or teenagers from previous marriages. Communication in these cases must be extremely clear and consistent to avoid conflict within the family unit. I have seen families grow and mature emotionally, just as I have seen families fall apart. Going back to the previous chapters, the emotional intelligence of each of the family members is key in order for them to communicate effectively and grow in all areas of their lives.

Identifying your priorities and understanding them as a couple is an extremely important role. Communication is key to avoid conflicts and maintain *harmony* in the home. On many occasions I have been able to share with families where they manage to serve in a way that they grow physically, emotionally and spiritually.

Thus, creating a healthy environment and citizens of the world who bring value to others.

Identify and create common plans

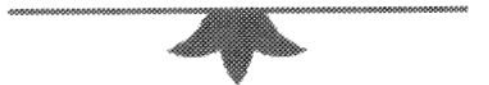

Personally, I believe that in order to achieve the balance we need, it is necessary to identify and plan together what is the most important strategy after communicating effectively. Identify projects where all members of the family can collaborate and participate. For me, this has been a very important strategy.

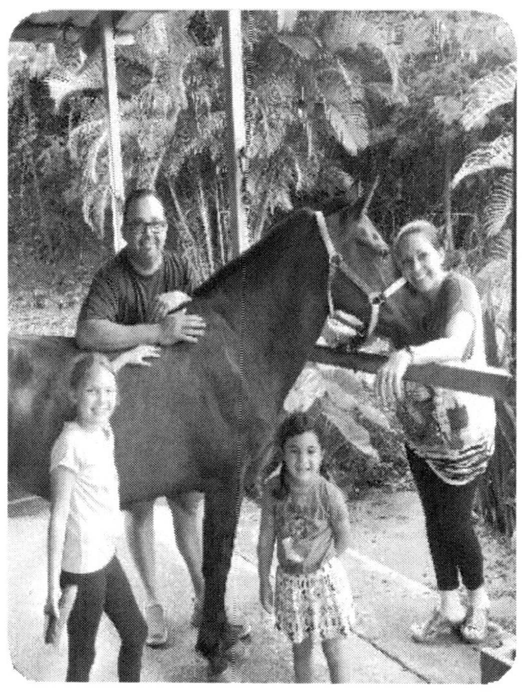

Sometimes, we all want to do different things and it is impossible to commit to each one of them. Therefore, having good communication and some common projects will allow the family to spend more time together. Likewise, I assure you that this will strengthen family ties. And how is this done??

Create a plan where everyone has a role and make sure everyone's roles are well defined. Even my little girl, Valeria, knows her role in each of our projects. We, as a family, volunteer in an equine therapy program for children with special needs. In fact, I am an instructor in that program and my husband, who also loves horses, although not an instructor, has learned various ways to help the children we serve in this program.

Serving this population not only fills our hearts but has taught us to be empathetic to these families who have children with disabilities. Raising children with disabilities is extremely challenging. Therefore, these hours that we as a family serve has given us the opportunity to offer a helping hand to people who need it so much. My daughters have changed. They show compassion to their classmates who have some type of disability, whether physical or mental. Doing chores and activities with Victoria and Valeria has taught them to be noble and patient children. Most of all, they, Mike and I enjoy the satisfaction of serving others.

Make a commitment

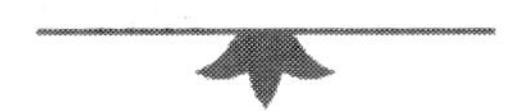

Decide how you can serve, try to include your family and get involved. It is more difficult to leave a volunteer position

when we are personally committed to the people who need our help. During my workshops I ask participants what kind of volunteer work they do or how they are serving the community. They look at me as if I am speaking to them in an unknown language. They don't even know what I'm talking about. Sad, isn't it? You may be an extremely busy person. However, in today's world, the busiest and most successful people are committed and take the time to serve, in some way or another, the community.

Serving adds value to your life. It makes you feel useful, because you bring value to others. So, don't forget to take time out of your schedule to commit to some social commitment.

Learn to say NO

If you are that talented and generous woman, people will come to you and ask for more help than you can give. Be careful! If your purpose in life and priorities are clear, there will be times when you have to say, "No". Saying, "I can't" to someone is not offensive. It is no reason for anyone to be offended. Don't forget the saying, "He who grasps too much, grasps too little" or, "It's better to do one thing well than many things poorly." If the place you are in does not respect your "no", it is a place where you should not be serving. They usually get upset because they don't understand the sacrifice and value of your services.

Serve with love

Finally, serve with love. Serving with love is the primary strategy for achieving *homeostasis* in your social role. There is nothing above or superior to love, love and be loved. Love is the best tool to experience satisfaction, contentment and peace. Love is the key to achieving our purpose in life. Without love it is not worth serving or assuming any social role. It would be a total waste of talent and time. If there is no love in what you are offering to others, don't do it. Reflect and evaluate all that we have discussed. Consider your purpose and start over.

FINAL THOUGHTS

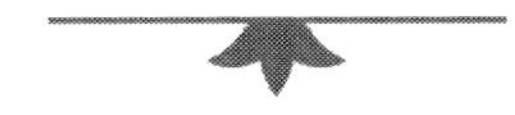

What a joy to see that I am at the end of this book! It has been a long, but highly positive and transformative process. As I have shared with you my knowledge, my way of looking at life, and my personal experiences, I have been able to understand myself and others more. I have grown in many areas of my life, especially during this pandemic caused by COVID-19.

Both you and I have faced great difficulties. We have had to adapt to a new reality. Being at home with the children all day has been challenging. Losing jobs has caused stress in families. We have felt vulnerable and the way we look at life has changed. We are different and we will never go back to the reality we once lived in. And what should our attitude be in the face of all this? "Para'lante!" as they say in my homeland of Puerto Rico. "Backwards, not even to gain momentum". Both you and I, we have to say to all these ailments and calamities, "No!"

How can we pull forward? We can get ahead by doing everything we can to live balanced lives; in other words, by achieving physical, emotional and social homeostasis. How? By putting into practice strategies that increase our bodily, emotional and social intelligences. Yes! We have to become smarter than ever. If living balanced lives was and is essential in normal times, how much more so when we are going through difficult times. We matter! We have significant roles in our families, careers and communities. To be effective we must first take care of ourselves and that care can only be achieved through total balance. I would like your permission to give you some tips that will help you emerge victorious from this global crisis.

The first is that you love others. No matter how far apart physically apart, love has no barriers.

Demonstrated love transcends distance. There is much you can do with your loved ones even if you have to keep your distance to protect us physically. Simply be concerned for the welfare of others. Do acts of charity especially for those who are suffering. You may have noticed by now that indifference, selfishness and lack of good manners reign in our society. People tend to think only of themselves, their own welfare or how to survive, even if they do so at the expense or over others. But you are different because loving others is, or should be, one of your priorities.

The second thing I advise you never stop tithing. Tithing is, or means, 10% of your financial income, talents and, above all, time. Your tithes are the first fruits of your blessings. You can give your tithes to the church where you congregate or the association dedicated to humanitarian service to which you belong. In other words, give 10% of your time, talents and money to a religious or secular organization that is dedicated to meeting the spiritual, emotional and social needs of your community. When you tithe from what God has given you, you serve humanity and refuse to be part of the collective self-centeredness. Tithing is a way of serving your neighbor.

The third thing I would advise you to do is to spend time with others, especially those who are ill, lack the resources to support themselves or simply live in loneliness. What has bothered me the most in this pandemic is how far away people became. For women it is particularly difficult because we are very social and enjoy spending time with family. We touch, hug and kiss to teach, show appreciation or reach out to others. This pandemic has negatively impacted our natural way of relating to each other. But there you are! Find ways to minimize this distancing. Make calls, send text or voice messages. Communicate through social media. Use apps like WhatsApp, Zoom or Skype to communicate face-to-face - it doesn't matter! The important thing is that you show the love you have for each other in the best way possible.

In short, both you and I can make history during these times. You are not like everyone else!

If you have read this book and guide it is because you want to grow, reach your goals and achieve your purpose in life. You have already learned how to achieve a state of physical, emotional and social homeostasis. I assure you that now, more than ever before, you are ready to reach your full potential and be a blessing to others. I conclude by asking you, what are you doing to make a difference in the world we live in today?

VOICES OF INFLUENCE

Here to close this, my first book, I leave you with the voices of women who influence my life in various ways.
I asked them: How do you define a balanced woman? These are their answers. Listen to what resonates between them. As there are common and key factors. As you read, take note and put it in perspective of everything we've discussed. At the end, I've created your own space for you to share What does being a balanced woman mean to you now? I've provided you with an email where you can share your photo and response. We would love to share it later on our pages.

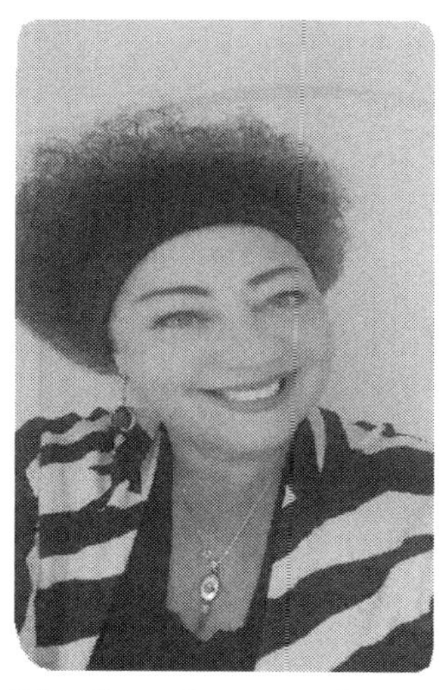

Dra. Lourdes Allen

Wife, mother, author, consultant and public speaker

Women, especially those who have immigrated to the United States, have left their homelands, cultures, families and all that was familiar, to achieve a better quality of life. They and I have faced many immeasurable challenges.

What sacrifices we have had to make! However, all those sacrifices would have been in vain without the blessing of a balanced and well-balanced life. In other words, a state of physical, emotional and social homeostasis is essential to achieving our goals and improving our quality of life wherever we live.

For me, women who have achieved a state of *homeostasis* are those who, despite the challenges they face in life, are able to maintain the balance or equilibrium needed to fulfill their multiple and complex responsibilities in the family, professional and community arenas.

In my 65 years of life, I have learned that the balance we crave and need is only achieved with abundant physical, emotional and social health.

Through this book, we have learned with Dr. Myrelis Aponte that the health we need so much to live balanced lives is achieved by developing our physical, emotional and, therefore, social intelligence. In other words, we have no choice but to become smarter. Period and that's it!

What I have enjoyed most about this book is the hope I have received. I believe and clearly see that achieving my purpose in life, and succeeding in all the roles I play, depends not only on God but also on myself. I can do it and you can do it if we really put our minds to it.

Thank you, Dr. Myrelis Aponte Samalot for sharing with us the need to live balanced lives and, above all, the strategies to achieve it.

Dra. Anitza San Miguel

Wife, mother, scientist, educator and coach

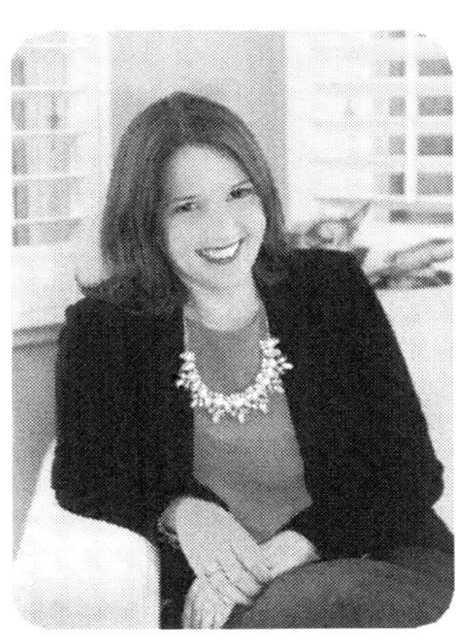

From my perspective and experience, a balanced woman is one who recognizes that she is imperfectly perfect. I am a perfectionist, I accept that.

With time (and experience) I have learned that I am not perfect and that there are areas in my life that I need to continue to develop. Disorder and chaos come into my life at the least expected time.

I remember my first years of marriage, before my daughter was born. My house was perfect, everything in order, picked up and in its place. When the light of my eyes, my daughter Andrea, was born everything changed. She completed me. She taught me that I am imperfectly perfect. She teaches me every day to focus and be present at all times. The collected house took a back seat, as the priority was my daughter and my husband.

Then, I started working full time and added more chaos to my life.

As I began to advance in my career the time became less and less. Over the years I learned that the reality is that time is the same: 24 hours.

I learned to manage myself. We talk about "managing time". The truth is that we cannot manage time. We can only manage me. It took me a while to recognize that at times toys were going to be all over the house. The kitchen was not going to be picked up. What did I learn? I learned to be in harmony with myself, my daughter and my husband. I learned that I can try to achieve balance, but what I really want to achieve is harmony.

I've had times in my life where I haven't been able to give 100%. I have given 75%. You know what? 75% is better than 0%, better than nothing. And that's okay. We women wear many hats... we are daughter, mother, grandmothers, nieces, friends, wives, sisters, businesswomen, sisters-in-law, mothers-in-law... Let's learn to be unique! I don't know about you, but I am imperfectly perfect.

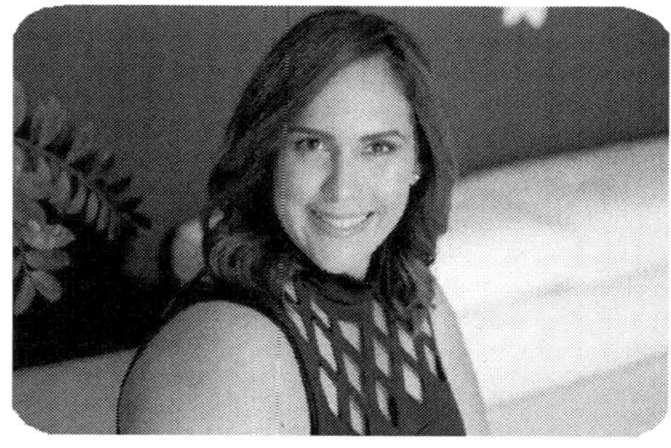

Ing. Lynda Vázquez

Wife, mother, engineer and businesswoman

I thank my friend, Dr. Myrelis Aponte for the opportunity to address women.

Thanks to Desarrollo Vital because it is an excellent tool to empower women all over the world.

Today the lifestyle of a woman has a very heavy role that only by the grace of God we can handle. I am a Latina, businesswoman, mother, engineer, wife, community servant, daughter and all these roles we live daily with a balance between God, family and work. Who gives us the balance? Well, faith, a positive attitude and being grateful help us to have a balanced life.

Gratitude must be practiced daily. That is why I am grateful for the good and the not so good. That way of living fills me with life and that gives us balance because everything has a purpose in life.

Women have an inner light that stands out anywhere in the world. That inner light comes from a Supreme Being who is the one who opens your doors through the gratitude you give daily. Practice and you will see a difference in your life.

It is in my heart to tell you with love that this Supreme Being wants to meet you and has open doors for you. His name is God. We are blessed to bless. I wish you much success in your lives. May God bless you all.

Dra. Laura Trinidad Olivero

Wife, educator and clinical psychologist

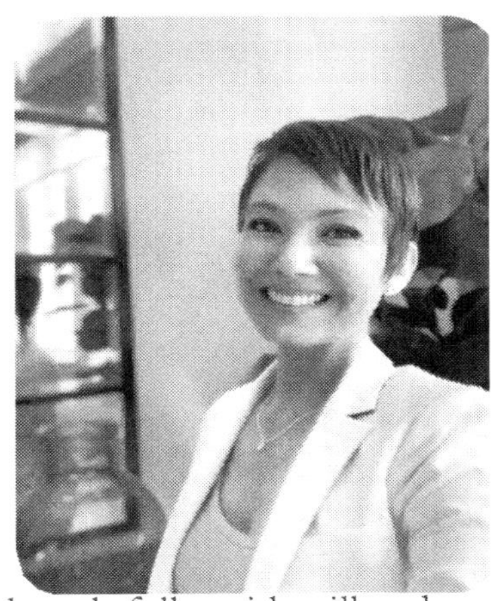

A balanced woman knows who she is. She knows who she is because she knows what distinguishes her, she has an identity. She recognizes her virtues and seeks to develop those areas for improvement. Her balance comes as a result of having her values clear. To have clear values is to take care and lead a life based on what is important to her. A balanced life is not a product of luck or coming from a good family or community; these things may influence, but they do not determine. To live with balance is to live deliberately. It is living thoughtfully, with will and purpose.

A balanced woman is wise. She not only distinguishes between right and wrong, but between good and better. She recognizes her limits and those of others. She knows when to say yes and when to say no. A balanced woman learns from her history and forges her future. A balanced woman lives in the present, visualizes her future and takes firm steps to make her plans come true.

To be a balanced woman is not to be perfect, it is to be the best of herself every day. This is not an easy task, but the possibility of discovering what she is capable of achieving and being able to impact others is the dynamo that drives her. A balanced woman is a whole woman, she is not lacking in any part, because she integrates her emotions, her thoughts, her physicality and her spirituality; her transcendence.

A balanced woman dreams, laughs, cries, fights, falls and gets up. She does not live without fears, she uses them to discover the unknown. A balanced woman defies stagnation, harbors change and lives in the present with expectation.

Arq. Mara Torres León

Wife, architect, artist and businesswoman

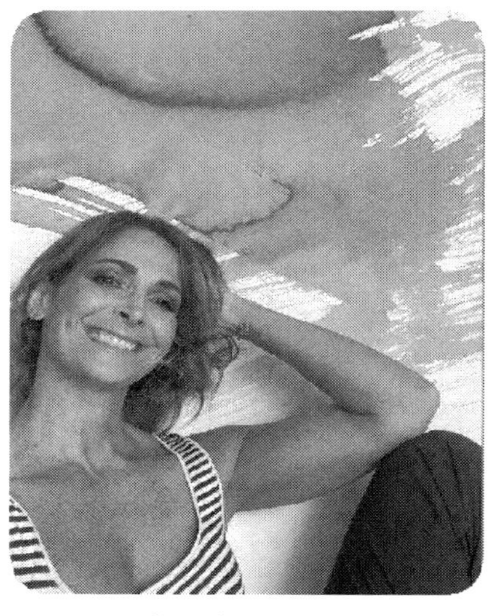

Emotional intelligence is a great virtue that some people have to know how to control their emotions in the most difficult moments. However, through the years and multiple situations that arise in this wonderful journey called life, as a woman I have discovered that one of our greatest qualities is the ability to be balanced within the chaos.

The roles we accept in society can often become repetitive, exhausting, intense and wonderful. To be balanced is to be able to look at our situations and emotions head on, accept them and face them, not suppress them.

Women know that changes are not necessarily bad and we identify our emotional and physical needs to share them with others. We give ourselves permission to accept criticism, and let failure become a source of learning.

We recognize that every experience has a lesson and this allows us to welcome changes that may arise, even though they may prove to be complicated later on. We are more confident than ever in who we are, what we are worth and our purpose to serve, help and impact the lives of many.

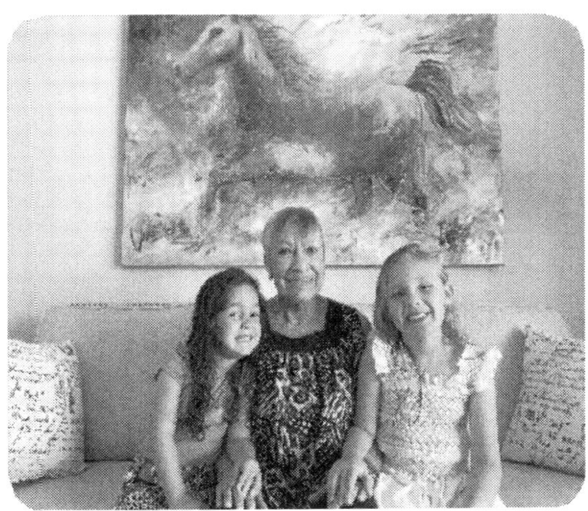

Myrna Samalot Pérez

Wife, mother, grandmother and administrator

Starting from the premise that we are categorized as "women", I think this idea gives us a balm of motivation to overcome ourselves and accept ourselves as we are. Starting with self-love, followed by love for others.

When we manage to love, recognize and accept ourselves, we create a responsible environment of empowerment, growth and respect. Despite being socially marked, we are able to demonstrate that our abilities go beyond gender.

Based on the maturity I have and having the privilege of being a daughter, wife, mother and grandmother, knowing from my youth the effort and sacrifice of carrying a family on my shoulders, I can describe a balanced woman as one capable of creating a realistic self-concept by recognizing her abilities and limitations, loving and valuing every beautiful moment and overcoming any negative feelings. Both you and I must adapt and adjust to change and fight tirelessly.

Be willing to receive new ideas, without forgetting your own. Know how to value the simple things in life.

The key to balance is based on recognizing that everything has a reason for being and no matter how difficult and how situations around us change, we must be certain that everything has a purpose and happens in a perfect divine order. It is a matter of looking for the positive side of every situation.

Today, I can see that a balanced woman in the greatness of my mother, in the strength of my daughter and in the dreams of my granddaughters, and in me as the proud grandmother of Victoria and Valeria, daughters of my beloved Mike and Myrelis.

Yeidra Rivera García

Wife, mother, leader and educator

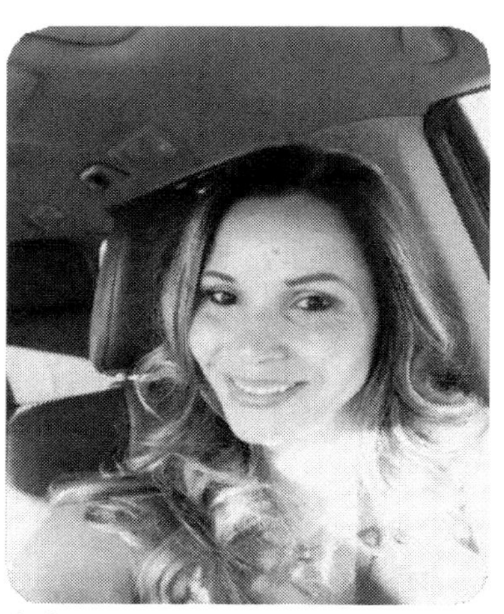

A balanced woman is one who acquires new disciplines or habits to empower herself in any circumstance. In life we will have to face and overcome many things. Only those women who achieve balance will be successful in all areas. I have learned many things throughout my life. The first is to be patient, sometimes we want things fast, but sometimes it is necessary to go through a process that leads to gain experiences, in which we acquire wisdom.

The second is not to be so demanding or to be perfect, because it causes a lot of pressure and frustration. I learned to see the simplicity of life and to live in the simplest but most meaningful way. Family time is very important, as you create memories and establish unbreakable bonds with the ones you love. It is very important to take time for you as a woman, to take care of your health, because sometimes we give so much that we wear ourselves out. If we are alert to our body and we feel uncomfortable, we must stop. Taking care of ourselves and eating well will give us the energy and health we need to keep going.

Taking time for ourselves helps us to balance ourselves and keep going.

For me, the most important thing is to prioritize God in everything we do. I come from a dysfunctional family and suffered a lot in my childhood. Today I can see the difference when you put God first. I have had to change habits to achieve a balance. It is not easy, but it can be done with perseverance, good decisions, good attitude, faith, organization and writing down your goals will lead you to the balanced and successful life you are looking for.

Elba L. García Pastrana

Executive, wife, sister, grandmother

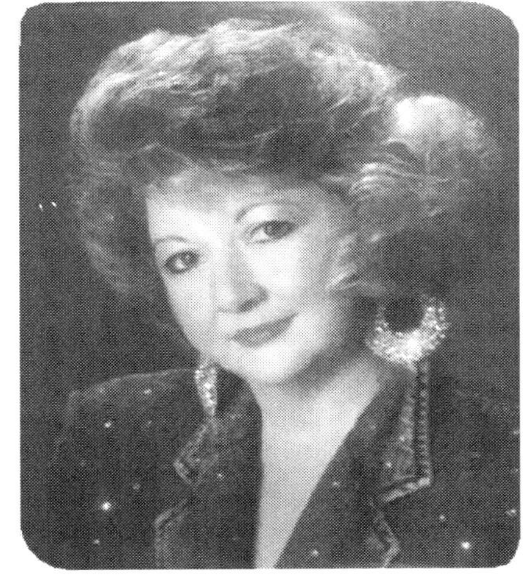

The first thing that comes to our mind when we hear the word "balance", is a thin rope, where one body is on it, with one foot in front of the other with their hands outstretched looking for that balance so as not to fall.

So, when we decide to keep walking, we think that's the way to solve our lives. Our dreams seem to be on that fine line.

That's the way our life is since we are born. We cry to be taken care of, whether it is hunger, pain, sleep or dampness. Though our life be with riches, poverties, joys, despair or fatigue, we have to move forward on that rope called balance and along the way we raise our arms to keep ourselves in balance.

But I tell you, life without balance is not possible to reach our goals. It is useless to have great goals if we are not able to put them into practice. We have lived a diversity of experiences but we must move forward along that rope called life. Maintaining that balance is essential for our family, be it mother, father, husband and children, as well as our dreams.

There is a thought of a great Puerto Rican man named Ramón Baldorioty de Castro: "if when I get out of prison, I don't find men to follow me, I will turn to women".

It is amazing how strong and balanced we are. Seek balance, it is within you.

Finally, I share with you that courage is not the absence of fear, but the triumph over it. The courageous woman is not the one who does not feel fear, but the one who conquers fear. That is evidence of being a balanced woman.

Mariel Sofía González

Wife, educator, counselor and businesswoman

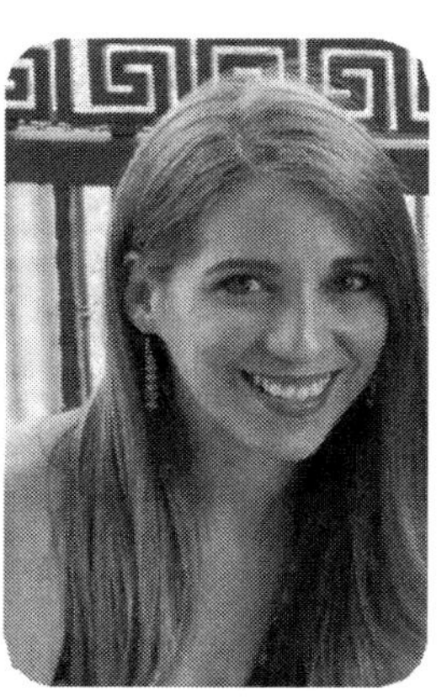

There is so much to discover. So much to learn, to overcome, to experience. Every step makes a difference. Every step has an impact, the extent of which we will not always understand.

Every decision made has its effects. I admire those who courageously make positive decisions, even if they are not necessarily the most common.

Decisions that have impacted second and third generations. We would like to think

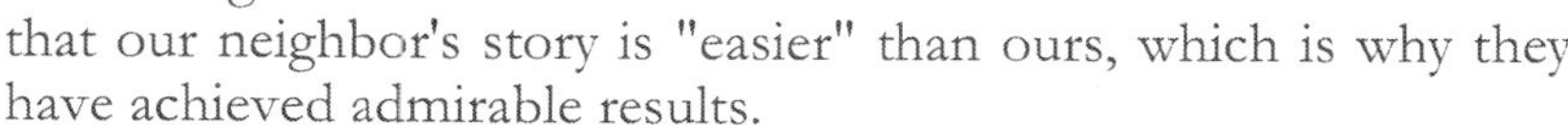

that our neighbor's story is "easier" than ours, which is why they have achieved admirable results.

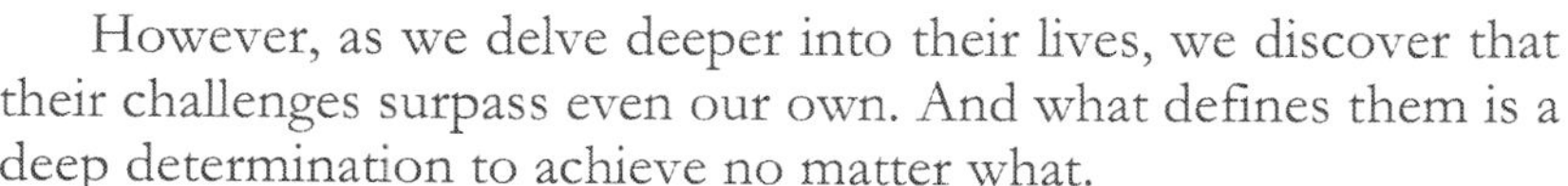

However, as we delve deeper into their lives, we discover that their challenges surpass even our own. And what defines them is a deep determination to achieve no matter what.

They are people who have believed and stuck with it until they achieve their goals and dreams. They have a deep hunger and desire to grow. To claim the blessings that are for everyone by divine inheritance. Perhaps, and most certainly, you are one of those people.

You are writing a success story every day. And if the path you are on today does not lead to the realization of that victory story, have the confidence and courage to begin a new direction. Keep moving forward. Don't give up.

Resume with more strength than ever. Look for alternatives, believe, follow and walk. Recognize your courage. And take flight.

If you fall, get up. If you cry, dry your tears. If you doubt, seek strength in your most cherished dreams. Renew yourself in the love of God. Persist. Don't try. Do it! Why not you? Why not me? Why not now?

FAREWELL

You are the difference. Through the lines of this book, I hope to have provoked curiosity to learn. In this way you will be able to develop, grow and thus transform yourself into a Latina woman who has achieved balance in her physical, emotional and social life. My greatest wish is that from now on you will seek a continuous state of homeostasis. There you will find harmony in all the roles you play in life.

I have spoken to you of love, I have spoken to you of service, and I have spoken to you of commitment. It is up to you to achieve the harmony you so desire. Remember, every decision you make will bring you closer to or further away from your purpose in life. I don't want to say goodbye, let alone close this book, without reminding you that you don't have to do it alone. There are mentors and coaches who can support you on your way to family, professional and social balance and harmony. In Desarrollo Vital https://desarrollovital.com/ we are here to support you on your way to homeostasis.

Through this book and guide, I have focused on the three letters: BGS that represent, **Body, Growth** and **Sharing**. I hope that in this new journey you will learn - first and foremost - to love yourself.

Take care of and respect your body! Grow in all areas of your life. Don't limit yourself, but expand. And finally, share with others the love you have for yourself and what you have learned in your growth. Don't live life for the sake of living. Give to others, become a leader and, above all, leave a legacy. Well, that's it, blessings to you, my friend!

Now is your turn!

After reading this book Homeostasis; how do you define being a balanced woman? If you want to share it you can send it to: dramyrelis@desarrollovital.com, I would love to see your exercise.

Your Name:

Your Photo:

ABOUT DR. MYRELIS APONTE

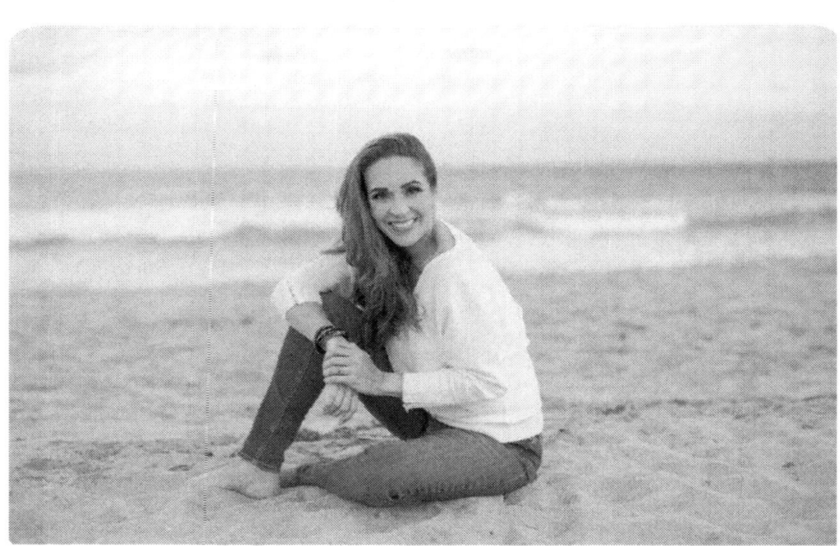

She was born into a middle-class family in Puerto Rico. Myrelis, quickly learned that education was the means to achieve and reach her goals. This led her to complete her Bachelor of Science degree and continue her graduate studies at the doctoral level.

From a very young age she held leadership roles. She led groups in school and was always physically active, excelling in dance, gymnastics and swimming. She grew up in a military school, so discipline and order were part of who she is today.

During her university years, she was also part of student and professional organizations' boards.

At the age of 16, she began to learn sign language and this was a passion that would take her in new directions. In 1998, she decided to go to the United States to pursue her master's degree at Gallaudet University. This university is unique in the world, as it specializes in studies related to deaf people. There she completed her degree in counseling with a specialization in deaf and hard of hearing people.

She decided to stay in the United States, now to work and overcome one of the biggest linguistic and cultural challenges to achieve her professional goals. There she became part of the mental health counseling team at the Model Secondary School for the Deaf in Washington, D.C.

She returns to Puerto Rico now to complete her doctoral degree in Clinical Psychology at the Ponce School of Medicine (now Ponce Health Sciences University). She then accepted an internship position in clinical neuropsychology at New York University Hospital in the Comprehensive Epilepsy Center. There she was responsible for developing protocols for the Hispanic population and earned recognition from the Hispanic Mental Health Association of New York.

In 2006, Dr. Myrelis Aponte Samalot returned to Puerto Rico as Associate Professor of the Ana G. Méndez University System. One of her goals was to be able to impart the knowledge and experience acquired. She developed the first university program for sign language interpreters. She also worked on important proposals, curricula and promoted the profession of interpreters on the island.

Dr. Myrelis also maintained a private practice in clinical neuropsychology and consulting offering workshops and conferences in and outside of Puerto Rico. Her clinical experience spans private and public sectors.

She is certified by the National Board of Certified Counselors and Coaches and is part of the National Register of Health Psychology. She is also certified as a **speaker, workshop leader, motivational speaker and coach** by the John Maxwell Team, Empowered Living, FEMA and ACER, among other certifications. She is also a certified therapeutic riding instructor. She is currently a national and international speaker on various topics such as neurolearning, brain health, communication, leadership, emotion management, team transformation, crisis management, among many others. Her energetic and interactive style provokes introspection and transformation of the human being. Her greatest passion, pleasure and purpose is to work with the realization of the dreams and goals of enterprising men and women.

Dr. Myrelis Aponte loves to share her talents everywhere she can reach. You will find her in many stages around the world.

Certifications

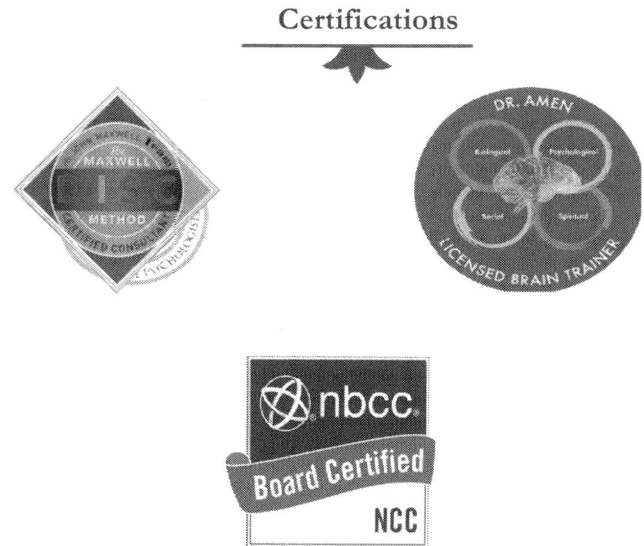

Made in the USA
Columbia, SC
17 November 2022

70826277R10080